HOMEOPATHIC REMEDIES

HOMEOPATHIC REMEDIES

FOR PHYSICIANS, LAYMEN AND THERAPISTS

David Anderson, M.D. · Dale Buegel, M.D. · Dennis Chernin, M.D.

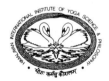

Himalayan International Institute
Honesdale, Pennsylvania

ISBN: 0-89389-037-5

Copyright 1978
Second Printing 1979

HIMALAYAN INTERNATIONAL INSTITUTE
OF YOGA SCIENCE AND PHILOSOPHY
Honesdale, Pennsylvania 18431

Special thanks to all those who have helped.

Table of Contents

Homeopathic Remedies

Introduction

This book was written to answer a need.

It has been many years now since Swami Rama established the Himalayan Institute in the Northwest suburbs of Chicago. Its lectures and courses on Yoga, relaxation, meditation, biofeedback and nutrition created in a growing number of people in this area a sensitivity to the needs of the body and an awareness of how to foster and maintain a state of natural good health. To the many people from all walks of life who attended the programs of the Himalayan Institute it became increasingly important to find ways of managing their health problems that would capitalize on what they had learned. They wished to minimize the use of drugs and surgery and when possible to restructure their habits of diet, exercise and thinking so as to eliminate the roots of disease and gradually and naturally restore genuine health. So there grew out of the Institute our therapy programs established to serve these people who had developed a sense of preventative medicine and a need for methods of treatment which are compatible with a balanced life and a clarity of consciousness. The Institute had created, in effect, a community which demanded a kind of health care geared not merely toward the relief of crisis and the alleviation of pain but aimed toward a rebalancing of the total functioning of the person.

It has been my privilege to help create a health care system designed to serve this enlightened community. It has attracted patients who are sincere, motivated and creative in their approach to working on their health and who are willing to seize the opportunity offered by their "illness" to learn more of themselves and to grow in health—physically, emotionally, psychologically and spiritually. It has been gratifying to see this medical facility expand and the demand for such services increase at a surprising pace. In the meantime it has been our pleasure to offer training in these techniques to physicians, nurses, clinical psychologists, social workers, etc. from around the country, attracting some of the most talented, sincere and promising young professionals.

Our major clinical work is centered on the unravelling and treatment of chronic health problems. Among the tools we found most useful was the Homeopathic Remedy, the prescription of which demands years of study and training if it is to be used to correct deep-seated constitutional disorders. Yet one of the cornerstones of our approach was, from the beginning, to encourage our patients and students to be creative and independent and to learn to manage minor crises on their own.

Therefore we gradually came to supply our

better-schooled patients with small kits of the less deep-acting homeopathic remedies to use at home for routine treatment of minor aches and ailments. Eventually it became necessary to offer a training course in the use of these remedies and requests for more detailed information on them and on other methods of managing health problems in the home grew. It was left to the energy and enthusiasm of three of the most outstanding of the young physicians who have come through training programs here at the Institute, Drs. Anderson, Buegel and Chernin, to systematize the knowledge that had been gained through years of experience and to offer it in such a way that it can foster the working relationship between the patient and the physician. They have provided a very practical book which not only will serve as a concise introduction to the subject of Homeopathy and to the use of tissue remedies, but also will put in clear perspective the home use of these techniques. They pass on to the reader guidelines for managing minor aches and pains and realistic advice as to when to consult a doctor, as well as a perspective on which prescribing, homeopathically, should be done by a physician who is highly trained. They have also included many of the helpful, common-sense measures for home use which are non-medicinal but which had been found through clinical experience to complement nicely the use of the homeopathic remedy.

It is with a special note of pride that I introduce this book to the public since it was my pleasure to initiate these three outstanding young physicians into the practice of homeopathy and to guide them during the many months that they labored to master its rigorous discipline. I owe them a debt of gratitude for putting this material before the public, a gratitude which I am sure many readers will share.

Rudolph M. Ballentine, Jr., M.D.
September, 1977
Glenview, Illinois

Section A

PRINCIPLES
OF HOMEOPATHY:
THEORY AND
TREATMENT

Principles of Homeopathy: Theory and Treatment

I. HOMEOPATHIC PHILOSOPHY AND THE VITAL FORCE

Homeopathy is a system of medicine that stimulates the individual to recuperate and cure himself. Within each person, there are natural mechanisms constantly attempting to correct imbalances, eliminate waste and maintain equilibrium. Homeopathic remedies are medicinal preparations which facilitate the process of self-cure and enable the organism to heal itself by following the laws of nature.

Homeopathy exemplifies universal order and parallels between human, mineral and vegetable kingdoms. Every entity, whether animate or inanimate, has a particular essence. In illness, certain individual characteristics and symptoms arise which, when seen together, form particular patterns. These patterns are also found in minerals and plants and can be matched with those qualities found in the ailing individual. That matching substance is selected as the remedy which helps put the individual back in balance and eliminate the disease.

Homeopathy is both an art and a science, using philosophical premises and scientific experimentation to help eliminate illness. As an artist, the homeopathic prescriber must be able to view the ailing individual as a whole and unique person, with particular idiosyncratic symptoms. Simultaneously, he must integrate all the subjective and objective facts into a functional whole to find the most compatible remedy. As a scientist, the prescriber must follow strict and empirically-proven laws to re-establish the health of the entire individual.

The principles of Homeopathy are ancient, dating back to India's Ayurvedic medicine and Greece's Hippocrates. In the late 18th century, Samuel Hahnemann, a German chemist and physician, began to re-verify and codify these concepts. He called this system of therapy Homeopathy. There are three fundamental laws upon which this system of healing is based. They are: (1) The Law of Similars; (2) The Law of Proving; (3) The Law of Potentization.

The Law of Similars reveals that the same medicine which cures a certain set of symptoms in a sick person will produce similar symptoms of that illness when given to a healthy individual. For example, as Hahnemann found, *Cinchona Officinalis* (Peruvian Bark), will stabilize fever and neutralize the pain of malaria-like symptoms. If, however, a well person ingests the bark over a period of time, he experiences the same fever and chills characteristic of malaria.

The Law of Proving involves the systematic verification of the first law. A certain number of healthy people are given a plant or mineral extract daily and symptoms and signs are recorded as they arise. Those symptoms which consistently show themselves are documented and called the "provings" of that medicinal substance. When similar symptoms and signs are seen in an ailing patient, the remedy with a corresponding proving picture is prescribed to maximize the person's response to the internal imbalance.

The Law of Potentization illustrates that the power of the remedy lies not in the amount or quantity but in its quality or subtle aspects. Potentization is effected mechanically by first diluting the remedy and then by forcefully shaking (succussion) or mixing (trituration). This process can be repeated from one to over one-million times. The result of this process is a medicinal substance whose properties are extremely potent, yet non-toxic, as there is very little physical substance to cause toxicity. For example, if enough crude arsenic is taken, death ensues; but if arsenic is first potentized, an effective and safe remedy results.

Fundamental to comprehending Homeopathic laws and the system's overall efficacy is the understanding of another concept called the "Vital Force." This is the energy which animates and drives the human being and which integrates the mind, body and soul of man. Similar concepts of energy, or force, are called *prana* in yogic philosophy and *chi* by the Chinese. Homeopathic remedies can act on this energy level. To better understand this concept, an analogy can be drawn between man and machine. Television is an empty box unless activated by an energy source. The "Vital Force" is like the electricity in the television, dynamizing the human being mentally and physically, just as electricity activates the TV circuits. When a malfunction occurs, disease sets in, and adjustments must be made on various levels. Most medicines act to replace the malfunctioning parts, only to temporarily palliate the problem; Homeopathic remedies, on the other hand, act to direct and realign the Vital Force itself, thus fine-tuning the essential balance within the individual.

II. SELECTION OF THE REMEDY

Proper selection of the remedy must be based on the whole person. All symptoms must be studied and matched with the remedy which produces the same symptoms in a healthy subject (the proving). All mental and emotional sensations and physical signs must be integrated into a complete picture. Consequently, a Homeopathic prescriber studies specific symptoms, as well as the total underlying essence.

Two categories of symptoms are of utmost importance in the evaluation of the case and selection of the remedy. These are: "Generalities" and "Modalities." These symptoms reflect the responses of the person as a whole rather than a specific symptom or characteristic. For example: What time of day does the problem worsen? Is the condition relieved by warmth or pressure? Are the symptoms aggravated by cold or movement? Did the nausea or sore throat begin after exposure to cold or dampness, or after overeating?

A third important category of symptoms for proper remedy selection is the mental and emotional state of the patient. To understand these, certain questions should be asked: Is the patient irritable and restless, or does he lie motionless, inert, wanting solitude? Does the condition correlate with increased crying? Did worry, grief, bad news, or fear precede the illness?

Peculiar, unusual and paradoxical symptoms often help in the final selection. Is a burning sore throat relieved by hot drinks instead of cold? Is the fever characterized by absence of thirst? Does the patient sip only small amounts of liquid even though very thirsty?

Generally, the symptom picture corresponds dramatically with that of the remedy. However, if no remedy seems to match the ailment, several considerations are pertinent. The history and observations may be inadequate, in which case more facts are needed. The illness may be only in its beginning stage, in which case the prescriber must wait patiently while new symptoms appear. Or, the illness may be complicated and severe, and the patient may be unable to relay his symptoms adequately, in which case a physician's help is needed. Another dilemma arises when some symptoms correlate well with a particular remedy while other symptoms are contradictory. In such a situation, selection of the remedy should be based on the most important symptoms, those within the three categories previously mentioned of "Generalities," "Modalities." and the mental/emotional state of the patient.

III. HOMEOPATHIC POTENCY

Homeopathic medicine deals with two basic categories of illness, the acute and also the chronic, constitutional illnesses. Acute illness can be subdivided into superficial, transient ones, and those that are life-threatening. This book deals with transient, acute illness. Malignant and chronic diseases that have deep-seated origins or are accompanied by physical degeneration must be handled by a trained physician.

Lower potency (see explanation of potencies given in following paragraphs) remedies which are discussed in this book are generally used in home prescribing. Higher potencies act more deeply on the Vital Force and must be used under the guidance of a physician. Of the several thousand remedies, approximately 30 are particularly useful for the layman in home prescribing. These are primarily derived from plant sources, although some are derived from minerals. (*Mercurius Sol* is potentized mercury).

Biochemics, sometimes called tissue salts or cell salts, are also used. These low-potency mineral preparations which were developed by Schuessler in the 19th century, help to re-establish inner balance (homeostasis) in much the same way as Homeopathic remedies do.

Preparation of a potentized remedy is a detailed and complicated process. Briefly stated, the first stage is to prepare a tincture of the selected plant by soaking it in a solution of alcohol and water for a certain length of time. Then one part of the tincture is diluted in 99 parts of alcohol and water and shaken many times, resulting in a "1" potency. One part of this mixture is mixed with 99 more parts of alcohol and water and again shaken, producing a "2" potency. For home prescribing, remedies made by repeating this process 6 to 30 times are used.

The biochemics (tissue salts) are made by mixing and grinding the crude mineral in ten parts of milk sugar. Then, one part of this is mixed with ten parts of milk sugar again. A 6X potency is produced after six of these steps.

Consequently, a homeopathic remedy or a biochemical preparation has little physical or molecular substance remaining. The shaking (succussion) and grinding (trituration) are of absolute importance since it is here that the subtle energies and Vital Force of the remedy are released. Although the quantity of physical substance is small, it has been empirically confirmed that the more triturations and succussions used in the preparation, the more potent the remedy.

IV. HOMEOPATHIC REACTIONS AND SECOND PRESCRIPTIONS

After the initial prescription, the interpretation of changes is very important. Observing reactions to the remedy is a complicated process, especially in chronic cases. For acute cases, however, observation is less confusing, and it is thus easier to decide whether the proper prescription has been made. The classic Homeopathic reaction in chronic disease is a slight aggravation of physical symptoms with simultaneous improvement in the internal mental state. Later, improvement of the physical symptoms also occurs.

In transient acute cases, however, the reaction more frequently seen is amelioration without an initial aggravation. Sometimes this improvement is instantaneous; but usually, and more long-lastingly, improvement occurs gradually. In both the above cases, the patient should be left alone since no further remedy is necessary.

A third type of reaction occurs when the patient gets better for a while but subsequently improvement stops or the condition deteriorates slightly. If the symptoms are still the same and the remedy matches, then repetition of the initial dose is indicated.

A fourth reaction occurs after giving a dose and seeing the symptoms change. In this case, a new prescription is necessary. In fact, some illnesses characteristically follow certain patterns. For example, when treating boils, the initial inflammatory (red, hot) stage requires *Ferrum Phos 6X*. Once swelling commences, *Kali Mur 6X* is necessary. Then *Silicea 6X* is needed to bring the boil to a head and promote drainage. *Calcarea Sulph 6X* is used to aid final healing once drainage has begun.

Another prominent example is found in treating upper respiratory illnesses where symptoms often change very quickly, often within a few hours. Initially, the prescriber may find *Aconite 30* fits the symptoms, but twelve to twenty-four hours later *Arsenicum 30* may be necessary.

Another reaction which is relevant to home prescribing is the one in which the patient fails to improve, or, in fact, worsens. Generally, this is due to incorrect remedy selection but may also be due to a more serious constitutional problem. The patient's symptoms may at first improve, but soon relapse occurs. Or, he may seem to improve physically, but emotionally and mentally he worsens. For example, the burning sore throat may be less intense after prescription, but the ailing individual feels agitated and irritable. Also, a reaction may occur in which the patient becomes progressively worse after the initial prescription. In these two cases, it is wise to wait and not give another remedy so the effects of the dose can wear off. Then the symptoms can be taken again to ascertain whether another remedy is indicated or if the physician is needed for further aid.

A common mistake in Homeopathy is overprescribing. The prevailing, faulty attitude is, "If a little doesn't cure it, perhaps a lot will." If the selection matches the symptoms, the Vital Force will be stabilized, and only the initial small dose is necessary. Overprescribing will cause much frustration by confusing the symptoms and may cause further aggravation of the ailment. One must treat Homeopathic remedies with respect since they can be deep and long-lasting in their effect. They are not dietary supplements. While generally safe, misuse and abuse can be harmful.

V. RECOMMENDED DOSAGE

Homeopathic remedies and biochemics are dispensed differently from allopathic prescription drugs.

Since the biochemics are of lower potency, more can be taken in a shorter time span. In more acute situations, three grains (3, 1-grain tablets or 1, 3-grain tablet) in one-half to one hour repetitions can be given although the usual dosage is every two to four hours. In acute cases, biochemics are usually taken for one to four days.

The higher potency Homeopathic remedies are often in the form of globules. Here, the liquid remedy obtained from succussion is dropped onto lactose (sugar globules) by the Homeopathic pharmacist. Two globules (1 - 2 grains) are given at one time and can be repeated to a maximum of three to four times. At least two to six hours should be spaced between administration of globules.

The amount given for a dose of Homeopathic remedies or biochemics should be cut in half for small children.

In the treatment of illness, 30th potency remedies should not be mixed, whereas 6X biochemics can be given while treating with other biochemics or higher-potency remedies. For instance, an individual with a white tongue and yellow discharge from the eye who is very weepy and has a tearful disposition may receive *Kali Mur 6X* and, an hour or so later, a dose of *Pulsatilla 30*. No allopathic remedies such as aspirin or acetaminophen should be taken with Homeopathic remedies. *Coffee tends to antidote many Homeopathic remedies and should not be taken while one is being treated homeopathically.*

There are four remedies recommended in this book which have special methods of administration. *Nux*

Vomica 30 and *Ferrum Phos 6X* should be taken at particular times of day. *Nux Vomica* should be given in the evening since it is most effective at this time. *Ferrum Phos 6X* should not be given after sunset since it has a tendency to create difficulty in getting to sleep. *Magnesia Phos 6X* is most effective when given with warm water. Twelve to twenty tablets are dissolved in one-quarter cup warm water and sipped at fifteen minute intervals. *Arnica 30* is a remedy often taken for traumatic injuries. Here is an exception to the previously-mentioned idea that remedies are to be taken only a few times. In cases of traumatic injury, doses of *Arnica* are often taken every two to six hours for a number of days to help the healing of bruised areas.

VI. CARE AND ADMINISTRATION OF REMEDIES

Tinctures are used externally, either as lotions or ointments; the higher potencies are used internally. Globules and tablets are dissolved on or under the tongue in a clean mouth, free of food, toothpaste, mouthwash, tobacco and other strong substances. The mouth should be rinsed with plain water before taking the remedy. These steps are taken so the medicines can be thoroughly absorbed into the blood stream. The remedies should be kept away from strong light, heat and especially from exposure to strong odors or scents such as camphor, menthol or incense. The tablets should not be handled. They should be shaken onto a clean piece of paper or kleenex, or into the cap of the container, and then transferred onto the tongue. Don't eat or drink 15 minutes before and after taking any of the biochemics. If more than one biochemic is to be taken at one time, they should be spaced *at least five minutes apart.* No food, drink or biochemics should be taken for one hour before and after dosage of the higher-potency Homeopathic remedies.

To prevent cross-contamination or antidoting, the remedies should be kept in the containers in which they are supplied, and not transferred to other containers.

VII. HOW TO USE THIS BOOK

Homeopathy is a profound science, and many years of study are required to understand its subtleties. Because of its consistency and easy usability, however, the average person can learn to prescribe homeopathically. Complicated knowledge of pathology and physiology is not necessary; rather, careful observation and common sense are the means for proper homeopathic home prescribing.

This book serves only as a guideline for the layman who wishes to assume more responsibility for his or her family's health. It provides a wholistic perspective to human health and takes the mental, emotional and physical manifestations of illness into consideration. Simple problems can generally be handled at home. Often, if treatment is properly given, there will be no need for a physician. This book, and the remedies suggested, however, must not be used as a substitute for the physician. Use discretion in the evaluation of any case. Problems which the family feels are too difficult to handle should be discussed with a physician.

When appropriate, dietary recommendations and other practical non-medicinal hints have been added. Often illness can be treated naturally, without medicines, by taking certain steps to aid the person's natural ability to recover.

The second section of this book is called, "The Clinical Repertory." In this section, categories of illness are listed alphabetically and appropriate Homeopathic remedies and biochemics are listed under each section. A brief description of each of the remedies' symptoms and characteristics are included.

The third section is called "Materia Medica." Remedies are listed alphabetically and described in more detail. It is a partial summary of the various uses which are listed in the Clinical Repertory. It is included so the prescriber has a more complete picture of the remedy, including mental and physical aspects. Most remedies in the Materia Medica have four subdivisions: (1) The "Generalities" provide an overall picture of the remedy; (2) the "Modalities" show what factors make the patient who needs that remedy worse or better; (3) the "Clinical Picture" subdivision represents areas of the body for which the remedy is useful and provides the prescriber with additional information for analyzing the case; and (4) the "Uses" subsection is a cross-reference to the Clinical Repertory (Section B) because it is a listing of the various categories of illness in the Clinical Repertory where the remedy was mentioned. *It is important that the remedy cover most of the symptoms of the patient.*

It is not necessary that the patient have all the symptoms of the remedy.

If two remedies seem to fit the symptoms of a sore throat, one should look at the Materia Medica to get an overall feeling of the essence of the remedy, in particular the generalities and the modalities. For example, *Bryonia* and *Belladonna* may both fit a particular type of sore throat and headache. By looking to the Materia Medica, one will discover that the patients who should receive *Bryonia* feel better lying down and want to be left alone; whereas *Belladonna* patients are characterized by excessive mental agitation, and lying down aggravates the ailment.

All the homeopathic remedies and tissue salts described in this book can be obtained from any reputable homeopathic pharmacy.

For home prescribing the authors recommend using the 6X potency for biochemics and the 30th potency for Homeopathic remedies.

It is important to remember that homeopathic remedies can help you only if used properly. With proper understanding and common sense, you can learn to prescribe successfully for your family.

GOOD LUCK AND GOOD HEALTH TO YOU!

Section B

CLINICAL REPERTORY

Clinical Repertory

I. ABDOMINAL PAIN

For successful treatment, the quality and character of the pain must be described and the general symptoms obtained. Abdominal pain may be a symptom of a serious medical condition, and if relief is not obtained with a well-chosen remedy, a physician should be consulted.

Biochemics

Ferrum Phos

Associated with menstrual periods and characterized by heat, flushing of face and rapid pulse.

Magnesia Phos

Useful in colic (pain) of the new-born; gas pain in the umbilical region with drawing up of legs and bending double. Used when there is amelioration by friction, warmth and belching;

also useful for colic in gout and gall bladder
attacks which come on shortly after meals.
In this case, a physician should be consulted.
Magnesia Phos 6X is most helpful when mixed
with 4 oz. warm water and sipped slowly every
15 minutes.

Natrum Phos

Good for colic of children with signs of acidity
such as vomiting curdled milk or cream, or
passage of green, sour-smelling stools;   this
patient also tends to have gas.

Homeopathic Remedies

Belladonna

Cases where relief is attained by bending forward; abdomen tender, distended, aggravated
by the least jar; skin hot, dry; often associated
with high fever, red, flushed face and extreme
mental agitation.

Bryonia

When the patient lies motionless and the pain
is made worse by the least movement, jar,
touch or pressure; also made worse by heat.

Chamomilla

Stomach is distended and gas is passed in small
quantities without relief. Often indicated in

teething infants. Better by application of local heat. With *Chamomilla* colic, one often has hot cheeks, red face, and perspiration preceding an attack; often follows a fit of anger; feels as if in some place the abdomen would break through.

Colocynthis

Gripping pains forcing the patient to bend double or press something into the abdomen. Patient is restless and may twist and turn to obtain relief. May be caused by undigested food, cold, or occasionally by a violent emotion such as anger. Some relief from hard pressure, unlike *Belladonna* and also from passage of gas. Very commonly used.

Ipecac

Gripping colic, like a hand clutching the intestines. Cutting pains across the abdomen left to right; particularly after acidic or unripe fruit. Worse by motion; better by rest. Associated with nausea and vomiting.

Nux Vomica

Caused particularly by overindulgence in food or stimulants (coffee, highly spiced food). Pinching, constrictive type of pains as if the intestines were being rubbed through stones. Abdomen generally hard and drawn in rather than distended, and sensitive to pressure. Worse on motion; better sitting or lying down.

II. ABSCESSES AND INFLAMMATION

An abscess is a form of inflammation which is localized to a small area rather than generalized. If generalized symptoms such as fever, headaches, lethargy, or multiple sites of infection are present, a physician should be consulted. An abscess (boil) generally starts as an area of redness followed by swelling and pain. As the fluid collects, pus is formed and gathers at the center of the abscess. This may break open and drain until the pus no longer forms and healing takes place. Once the fluid has started to collect, several measures are taken to help bring the boil to a head and facilitate drainage. The best method is to apply warm wet-packs to the area of the boil. A moist pack should be applied several times a day for twenty minutes.

It is important not to irritate the site of the boil by attempting to squeeze the pus out. This will cause the inner borders of the abscess to break and spread the infection inward, becoming systemic or generalized in nature. Except when wet-packs are applied, the site of the abscess should be kept dry, free from irritation such as clothing, and left open to the air as much as possible. One should not cover the abscess with non-porous material as this will not allow oxygen to reach the infection and may lead to a more serious infection called gangrene. If the abscess is draining, one should cover it with a porous material such as cotton gauze which will allow the site to breathe and yet soak up the drainage.

Biochemics

Calcarea Sulph

This should be given after the abscess begins to drain. It will aid the healing process of the surrounding tissues and should be given as long as there is drainage.

Ferrum Phos

This remedy should be used if there is evidence of a generalized inflammatory process occurring such as fever or multiple sites of inflammation. It should be used early in the course of an inflammation.

Kali Mur

Begin this remedy during the second stage of infection where there is swelling and pain but no pus formation. It should be continued even after the pus has formed if there is continued swelling and pain.

Silicea

If *Kali Mur* does not cause resolution of the swelling, then *Silicea* will help the pus form and the boil come to a head.   It should be given every two hours until the boil begins to drain and gradually tapered over a day or two as the congestion and swelling go down.

Homeopathic Remedies

Apis
Indicated in the early stages of abscess if it appears like a bee sting with shiny swelling of the parts, redness and stinging pain. Sudden appearance of the abscess and intolerance for heat, with worsening of the pain at the slightest touch.

Arnica
Itching, burning, eruption of small pimples or crops of boils. Sensitivity to touch. Skin may be black and blue and have a bruised feeling.   Abscesses and boils do not mature but shrivel and crop up again. The *Arnica* patient feels bruised and sore, boils occurring after injury.

Hepar Sulphuris
Sensitive to drafts and has unhealthy skin where an abscess may start from the least

scratch. Abscess appears with a small pimple which rapidly ulcerates and begins to enlarge. Later, it is a putrid ulcer surrounded by small pimples. There is extreme sensitivity to touch with pains being sharp and stabbing or sometimes prickly in character. It becomes worse from cold applications; better with warm applications. There is a tendency to bleed.

III. ASTHMA

The wheezing and difficulty in breathing of asthma is generally a manifestation of a more chronic disease which needs the treatment of a physician. Several measures, however, may help the patient during the acute attack. The patient should remove himself from the precipitant of the attack if this is known, such as certain animals, food, fabrics, types of dust, etc. In general, the person should try to relax, avoiding heavy exertion, cold air, and certain foods that may aggravate the mucus associated with the symptoms such as dairy products, sweets, meat, wheat, oats, and in some cases, barley and rye.

Biochemics

Kali Mur
Where the tongue is coated white and there is

white mucous which is hard to cough up.

Magnesium Phos

For spasmodic nervous asthma associated with a paroxysmal, dry, tickling cough and difficulty when lying down. Flatulence (gas) is also present.

Natrum Sulph

Generally used in chronic treatment rather than as a home prescribing measure. Attacks usually come on in the morning around four or five o'clock with a cough and expectoration (material coughed up) resembling egg white. Later expectoration is greenish and quite copious. There may be vomiting after eating. The patient is always worse in damp, rainy weather. Often indicated in asthma of children. The patient tends to have loose bowel movements on rising in the morning.

Homeopathic Remedies

Arsenicum

Time of attacks is generally just after midnight. There is a great deal of anguish and restlessness and fear of lying down because of feelings of suffocation. Associated with a dry, burning cough and with burning and soreness in the chest. There is little expectoration but, if present, is frothy. *Arsenicum* is often given after *Ipecac* during the course of an acute attack.

Carbo Veg

Usually comes on in the evening and is associated with long coughing attacks with soreness and burning in the chest. Worse in open air and after eating or talking. The patient is usually old and debilitated. Cough may be spasmodic with gagging and vomiting of mucus.

Ipecac

Again, there is great anxiety with sudden wheezing, shortness of breath, and a feeling of suffocation. There is a sensation of a great weight upon the chest. The burning pains of *Arsenicum* patients are absent. There is often a cough which causes gagging and vomiting. The cough is constant and the patient feels his chest full of phlegm, but none is brought up. The extremities are covered with cold perspiration.

Nux Vomica

Attacks of simple spasmodic asthma brought on by gastric disturbances. There is some relief by belching, and the patient must loosen his clothing. Patient is usually irritable and fiery and will feel a constricted feeling at the lower part of the chest. *Carbo Veg* also alleviates asthma through belching, but the *Carbo Veg* patient is generally elderly and debilitated, unlike *Nux Vomica.*

IV. BITES (See Injuries)

V. BLEEDING

For chronic bleeding tendencies, external or internal, the advice of a physician should be sought. For any local bleeding, direct pressure should be applied. If bleeding is profuse (such as from trauma) the person should be kept warm and moved if possible to a quiet, comfortable place. Medical attention should be sought as soon as possible.

Biochemics

Ferrum Phos
For bleeding internally or externally with bright red blood which rapidly clots. Also for vomiting of bright red blood, although in this case a physician should be sought.

Kali Mur
When the blood is black, clotted or tough. Possible vomiting of dark, clotted, thick blood. Nosebleeds of this type tend to occur

in the afternoon.

Homeopathic Remedies

Aconite
When the blood is bright red and there is panic as well as a thirst for ice water.

Arnica
Always given first if bleeding follows injury.

Arsenicum
Restlessness, shifting of position and marked exhaustion. These symptoms may indicate a large amount of blood loss, and a physician should be consulted.

Belladonna
Blood is bright red, feels hot and clots readily. The head is usually hot and the face red.

Bryonia
Blood is dark yet fluid and usually associated with nausea and faintness when attempting to sit up. There can also be headache. The condition is made worse by the least movement.

Carbo Veg
Bleeding which is associated with symptoms of collapse such as clammy skin and a great desire

for air. Can be a steady seepage of blood. These are symptoms of hypotensive shock, and a physician should be sought immediately.

Ipecac
Bleeding comes in gushes of bright red blood associated with severe nausea, dark bluish crescents below the eyes, gasping aspirations. Especially indicated if these symptoms are associated with nosebleed or hemorrhage from the uterus. Immediate medical attention should be sought.

VI. BRUISES (See Injuries)

VII. BURNS (See Injuries)

VIII. CHICKEN POX
Although this illness may present a very constant picture of physical signs, the constitutional or temperamental aspects of the case must be taken into account.

Biochemics

Ferrum Phos
Most useful biochemic for chicken pox. Used in alternation with the remedy indicated by the type of eruption on the skin. The homeopathic physician should be consulted in selecting additional tissue salts or higher-potency

homeopathic remedies which may be indicated.

Kali Mur
Should be taken as soon as eruptions appear, to help diminish scarring.

Homeopathic Remedies

Pulsatilla
Child mild, tearful and not thirsty.

Rhus Tox
If there is great restlessness of mind and body.

IX. COLLAPSE AND SHOCK

These are essentially the same conditions. The term shock is used more in connection with accidents and operations, and collapse in relation more to "medical" cases. The signs and symptoms of the conditions are ashen grey pallor, cold, clammy skin, rapid and weak pulse, restlessness and shallow respiration. Certain immediate measures should be carried out in cases of shock. The patient should be reassured and fear allayed. He should be kept warm with feet elevated. Homeopathic remedies are of value before medical help is available.

Homeopathic Remedies

Aconite
If fear is very marked, especially fear of death.

Arnica
When there has been injury or bleeding.

Carbo Veg
When there is great hunger for air, desire to be fanned; coldness, particularly of the knees; or cold breath.

X. CONSTIPATION

This is an indication of a more chronic process and, if persistent, one should see a physician. For temporary constipation, squeeze ½ lemon into 8 oz. of hot water with a pinch of salt and 1 teaspoon honey; drink in the morning just after rising.

XI. COUGH (See Respiratory Infection)

XII. CROUP

This is an acute infection of young children 2 to 4 years. It is rare under six months. It usually occurs at night, the child waking into paroxysms of breathlessness characterized by crowing inspiration, barking, metallic cough, husky voice and violent struggle for breath. The attack lasts one-half to three hours and then eases. It is apt to recur for two to three nights. Both child and parent are usually terrified, and this tends to aggravate the spasm.

Three remedies have been found of special value in this condition. The most applicable one should be given every two hours until improvement.

Homeopathic Remedies

Aconite

To be used in the beginning of an attack, especially if there is anxiety or restlessness and tossing about. Patient may have hot skin; coughing is dry, loud and barking without expectoration.

Hepar Sulph

Croupy-sounding cough, but with a certain amount of moisture. There may be enough looseness that the child will have choking fits. Pains tend to go from throat to ears, and there may be expulsion of pieces of membrane.

Spongia

Croup with dryness of air passages. Usually the third standard remedy following *Hepar Sulph*. Cough dry, barking; croup worse with inspiration and before midnight. Alleviated by eating and drinking, particularly warm drinks.

XIII. DENTITION (Teething)

Babies often have difficulty with restlessness and irritability when their teeth are coming in. Homeopathy can offer relief for children and anxious parents.

Biochemics

Calcarea Phos

Should be given in any disorder related to teething, such as diarrhea, vomiting, fever, etc.

Homeopathic Remedies

Chamomilla

Great sensitivity and irritability. Demands toys yet throws them about immediately; desire to be carried. Often thirsty, diarrhea, dry cough before midnight.

XIV. DIARRHEA

This is an acute or a chronic condition. The former will generally pass in its own time. If it occurs in children, one should be sure the child drinks enough so that he will not become dehydrated. In chronic cases, the physician should be consulted. In chronic diarrhea of children, the offending agent has sometimes been found to be aluminum in the food caused by cooking with aluminum pots and pans.

Homeopathic Remedies

Aconite
Diarrhea brought on by exposure to cold, dry wind or the result of fright.

Arsenicum
Severe, burning diarrhea resulting from taking tainted food and associated with vomiting, prostration, restlessness, burning and anxiety. Stools are scanty, brown, excoriating to the skin; pain with defecation. Desire for hot drinks.

Bryonia
Profuse purging, especially with taking cold drinks or when overheated. Stools are brown, thin and smell like old cheese. Even when there is little disturbance of the bowels during the day, there is often diarrhea as the patient gets out of bed in the morning. Person is irritable, lies motionless, and wants to be alone.

Chamomilla
Diarrhea associated with teething in infants

(see dentition).

Colocynthis

Frequent, jelly-like stools with colicky pains. Temporary relief from passing stool. Made worse by food or drink. Pains made better by drawing legs up and by firm pressure against stomach.

Ipecac

Green, frothy or slimy stools. Gripping pain around the navel. Associated with nausea and vomiting.

Mercurius Sol

Stool is green, bloody and slimy with pain on passing; "never-get-done" feeling. Often associated with chilliness and sick stomach. Worse at night.

Nux Vomica

From dietary indiscretion. Diarrhea alternating with constipation. Worse in morning and after large meal.

Rhus Tox

Diarrhea with bloody mucus; tearing pains down legs; extreme restlessness with fever.

XV. EAR PROBLEMS

Simple, acute earache is often from congestion due to colds which can respond quickly to the appropriate remedies. The ear should be treated with caution since inflammation behind the eardrum can also involve the throat and Eustachian tubes and can spread its infection to other structures in the head. If pain or drainage does not subside within approximately 24 hours, a physician should be contacted.

For foreign bodies in the ear, one should not attempt to dig them out manually. Sometimes gently syringing the ear with warm water (or sterile olive oil), approximately body temperature, will float the object to the surface and out of the ear. If any object is introduced into the ear, there is danger of perforation of the eardrum—especially when done by inexperienced hands.

Biochemics

Ferrum Phos

Burning, throbbing earache with sharp, stitching pain. Pulsation in ear and head, with beefy redness of eardrum. Drainage from ear may be bloody. Use for earaches after exposure to cold or wet conditions.

Kali Mur

For earaches associated with white tongue and swollen glands and throat. Cracking noises may be heard in the ears on swallowing or blowing the nose. Deafness from swelling. Congested nose. Right side is more affected than left.

Homeopathic Remedies

Aconite

Acute onset often after a chill or draft. Violent pain. May be better with application of local heat. Ears red, hot, painful, often affecting the left ear more.

Belladonna

Face is red, hot and dry; pain is aggravated by the least jarring. Digging, throbbing pain often on the right side; heat may give relief. Thirst is absent, even with fever present. Often associated with sore throats and swollen glands.

Chamomilla

Pain is worse by application of local heat. Child may be very cross and fretful. Child feels better if held. Pains are very severe—making the patient cry out.

Hepar Sulph

Stitching pain; often starts as a sore throat and spreads to the ear. Desire for ear to be warmly wrapped. Tenderness in the bone behind the ear. Peevish patient; nothing pleases him. Worse in the least draft. May start in left ear and spread to the right.

Mercurius Sol

Pinching, sharp pains in ear, often extending to cheeks and/or jaw. Made worse by lying in bed.

Pulsatilla

Brought on by being chilled after being hot, or after getting wet. Pain is worse from application of heat. Patient weepy, wanting attention and company.

XVI. EPILEPSY

One should consult a physician in the event of seizure. Immediate care should be provided to the patient to keep him from injuring himself. This may consist of holding a patient's arms and legs so that he does not fracture them by swinging them against something. Place the person on his left side or stomach. Care must be taken that the patient does not swallow or bite his tongue during the episode. To prevent this, something such as a wallet may be placed between his teeth. This should not be done forcibly, however, as it may result in fractured teeth. Consult physician immediately.

XVII. EYE DISORDERS

Most foreign bodies can be washed out of the eye using large amounts of plain water. If a sensation of a foreign body remains, one should evert the lid. The upper lid may be everted by placing a thin, round object such as a matchstick handle above the eye, below the eyebrow and bone of the forehead, grasping the eyelashes and pulling them upwards as the patient looks downward. If the object can be seen and it is not imbedded, the moist end of a kleenex can be used to gently brush the object away from the lining of the eye. If there is pain following the removal of the object, or some bleeding, rinse the eye with **Calendula** lotion and apply **Calendula** ointment to the margins of both the upper and lower eyelid.

In general for trauma to the eye, cover the eye with a clean, moist cloth. If there is bleeding, **Calendula** lotion should be used. For a black eye, **Arnica** may be used internally followed by **Ledum** if discoloration persists. For injury to the eyeball itself, after surgical operations, and from irritation from foreign bodies in the eye, **Aconite** (with Arnica) should be used. For direct injury to the eye, it is best to consult a physician. For chemical injury to the eye, the best treatment is rinsing with water—gallons of it! This is especially true if the substance which has irritated the eye was alkaline. Burns to the eye are best treated with rinsing with **Hypericum** lotion (mother tincture diluted with water approximately 1:20). This also may be used after the initial rinsing with a chemical burn. In addition, one of the internal burn remedies such as **Cantharis** may be used.

XVIII. FAINTING

When someone has already fainted, most cases may be treated by loosening the clothing, keeping the patient horizontal and providing him with fresh air. Often fainting can be averted by sitting in a squatting position either on a chair or on the ground with the knees up, placing elbows on the knees and hands over the eyes. If fainting tends to recur frequently, one should consult a physician.

XIX. FEVER

It is important to know how high the temperature is and to take the temperature frequently enough to determine whether it is going up or down. The temperature may be taken under the arm, under the tongue, or rectally. Keep in mind that normal body temperature is 98.6° F measured beneath the tongue. Temperature measured under the arm will be one degree lower than when measured under the tongue; temperature measured rectally will be one degree higher than when measured under the tongue. Fever is an indication that the body is responding to illness and it is important in the healing process. To further aid the body in cleansing, drink plenty of fluids such as vegetable broth, water, or hot water with freshly-squeezed lemon juice and a little honey. In general, more substantial food such as dairy products, sweets, and grains tend to aggravate the fever.

If the temperature is very high (103.5° F or above, measured under the tongue), one should begin sponging. This should be done with lukewarm water and should not be overdone. Start first by sponging only the forehead and face and observing the effect on the temperature. If the temperature drops to 102° or below, the sponging can be stopped. If more extensive sponging is required, the extremities and torso also may be moistened. Do not attempt to drop the temperature back into the normal range by sponging as this will merely suppress the fever.

Biochemics

Ferrum Phos

Dry heat felt in the face, throat and chest. Quickened pulse. Generally useful in all fevers. There may be a chill associated with the fever in the early afternoon.

Kali Mur

Thick, white coating on the tongue; the least draft of cold air will chill the patient thoroughly. Patient may sit near a fire and be adequately covered but still feel cold.

Homeopathic Remedies

Aconite

Anxiety and restlessness; dry skin; violent thirst; relief from sweating. Brought on by exposure to dry, cold winds or chilling of the body by overheating. Frequent chills. Patient tends to be young and robust, rather than weak and sickly.

Belladonna

May have violent delirium; throbbing pulsation in the neck. Skin is hot and burning; eyes red and glistening. May sweat profusely without relief. Little or no thirst.

Bryonia

Patient is made worse by movement and prefers to lie still. Faintness on rising; dry mouth and white, coated tongue. Cold, chilly sensations are predominant. Much thirst for large quantities of water at rather infrequent intervals. Can have intense headache always aggravated by least movement.

Gelsemium

Dull, sluggish, apathetic condition. Patient may be dizzy and drowsy. Fevers brought on by warm, relaxing weather. Absence of thirst.

Pulsatilla
Head feels hot but otherwise chilliness predominates; can have intolerably burning heat
at night. Thirstless fever with dry lips. Patient
usually very weepy and continuously desires
comfort.

XX. HAYFEVER

This is generally an indication of a chronic condition requiring a constitutional remedy rather than
acute treatment. There is a helpful technique in which
one washes the nasal passages with warm salt water.
The proper technique must be learned from an ex-
perienced teacher in order not to trap water in the
sinuses causing infection. In the meantime, several
of the biochemics or remedies can help.

Biochemics

Kali Mur
Sensation of swelling associated with white
coating on tongue.

Magnesia Phos
Take every hour in warm water during the day
and evening, particularly if troubles come on in
sultry weather and patient is stuffy during the
day, with pressed, short, anxious breathing.

Homeopathic Remedies

Arsenicum

Sneezing is violently painful, and there may be a tickle in one particular spot inside the nose, not relieved by sneezing. Profuse, watery discharge which burns the lips. Patient restless and worried. Made worse by changing weather.

Dulcamara

Eyes swell and water and then the nose runs, followed by the eyes watering again. Constant sneezing with stuffy nose. Worse in the open air and from dampness. Can arise from contact with newly-cut hay. Patient feels chilled when skin is actually hot.

Gelsemium

Eyes feel hot and heavy; tingling sensation in the nose with violent sneezing. Nose streams particularly in the morning and the discharge is excoriating. Throat dry and burning; swallowing can cause pain in the ears. Face is hot. Patient aches all over with limbs feeling heavy.

Nux Vomica

Prolonged distressing spells of sneezing. Nose is more apt to be stuffed at night. Irritation of nose, eyes and face, with face feeling as if it were close to a hot iron plate. Patient chilly.

XXI. HEADACHES

Headaches are most often a symptom of more chronic constitutional tendencies than an acute illness. They are a guide for the treatment of chronic conditions and should not be suppressed with pain killers such as aspirin or stronger chemicals. Some headaches have as precipitating factors excesses of living such as drinking, lack of sleep, poor diet, or constipation. These habits must be corrected rather than suppressing the symptom that results from this condition. While treatment for the chronic condition is being sought, several remedies can help the acute condition.

Biochemics

Ferrum Phos
Bruising, pressing or stitching pain caused from a cold or from heat of the sun. Pains are worse on stooping and moving. Pressing a cold object against the spot relieves the pain. Headaches are pulsating and worse on the right side. Patient may feel a rush of blood to the head. Often cannot bear to have the hair touched. Can be used to treat headaches following injuries to the head, especially after failure of

cure by *Arnica*—but in such cases, the physician should be consulted.

Magnesia Phos

Shooting and stinging pains, which are intermittent and come on suddenly. Relieved by warmth. Headache is worse in the occiput and can be constant while attending to mental labor. Especially useful in tired, exhausted, neurotic patients.

Homeopathic Remedies

Aconite

Sudden, violent headaches as if the skull would be forced out of the forehead, or as if the skull were constricted by a tight band.

Apis

Stinging pain like bee sting; head bent backward or bored into pillow; pain often occipital. Aggravated by heat, warmth. Alleviated by cold.

Arnica

For headaches after injury. If headache persists, consult physician.

Belladonna

Throbbing with violent shooting pains driving

the patient almost wild. Patient *cannot lie down*, nor can he bear light, drafts of air, noise or jarring. Pain is most often in frontal region on the right side. Patient has flushed face or dilated pupils. Better with warm wraps to the head, bending the head backwards, or firm pressure.

Bryonia

Bursting, splitting, crushing headache. On attempting to sit up, feels sick and faint. Drowsy, dry, peevish; hot, flushed face. Better lying down. Wants to be left alone and feels better staying motionless.

Gelsemium

Occipital headache associated with great heaviness of eyelids and limbs. Hammering at base of brain. Not thirsty. Aggravated by mental effort, heat of sun, tobacco smoke.

Ignatia

Often follows anger or grief; made worse by smoking; head feels heavy, worse stooping. Feels as if nail driven through it.

Nux Vomica

Splitting headache, as if a "nail were driven into skull"; nausea and sour vomiting. Wakes up with it or it comes on after eating. Aftereffects of over-indulgence in food or alcohol.

Pulsatilla

Periodic headache. Pressure, distension or throbbing; from eating ice cream, rich food or over-indulgence. Patient tends to cry.

Ruta

Headache after eye strain; eyes are red, hot, tired, especially after prolonged close work such as sewing or reading small print.

Sticta

Dull aching over forehead with a pressure feeling at the root of the nose (near eyes). Headache before nasal discharge begins.

XXII. HEMORRHOIDS

This is a symptom of chronic disease and is best treated by a physician. For relief of an acute attack, until help can be sought, apply **Calendula** ointment externally if the hemorrhoids are bleeding.

Biochemics

Ferrum Phos

Bleeding, bright red blood with a tendency to form a thick, soft mass.

Homeopathic Remedies

Nux Vomica

Large hemorrhoids with burning, stinging and constricted feeling in the rectum, as well as a bruised pain in the small of the back. Especially indicated in people who have sedentary habits or use stimulants. The itching hemorrhoids keep the sufferer awake at night. Relieved by cold water. Bleeding piles with constant urging to stool and a feeling as if the bowel has not emptied itself.

XXIII. HICCOUGH

Generally a self-limited condition, but for very obstinate cases causing long-standing soreness, use Magnesia Phos in warm water (see dosage section of Materia Medica).

XXIV. HOARSENESS

Generally a self-limited condition but may also accompany colds and/or some chronic diseases. One of the most important treatments for hoarseness is to rest the voice.

Biochemics

Ferrum Phos

Painful hoarseness of singers and speakers. Onset often due to drafts, colds, or wet conditions.

Homeopathic Remedies

Aconite

Good in the beginning of laryngitis, particularly in children. Often associated with fever, chills and dry skin. Also may have croupy cough (see Croup).

Arnica

Hoarseness from trauma or overuse, as in yelling or singing.

Carbo Veg

Painless hoarseness, particularly when brought on by exposure to damp evening air. Aggravated in moist, cool weather. Generally worse in the evening, although symptoms present in the morning as well.

Hepar Sulph

Patient very sensitive to slightest draft; often associated with exposure to dry, cold winds. A remedy for children, as well as singers. Especially good for chronic hoarseness in professional singers.

Ipecac

Also recommended for complete loss of voice from cold or congestion if associated with nausea and vomiting.

Rhus Tox
Hoarseness from overstraining the voice, or during influenza when bones ache.

XXV. INDIGESTION

Indigestion may be acute or chronic. For chronic diseases, consult a physician. The acute variety is generally due to overeating, eating too quickly and not chewing the food; eating too many different types or too many incompatible foods at the same sitting. Correction of eating habits will prevent the indigestion from occurring. Acute indigestion is generally self-limited. Emotional upset and mental stress such as anxiety, fear, anger, resentment, impatience and over-work also contribute significantly to this disorder. The remedies are only temporary. If such symptoms occur, take note of the emotional life as well as dietary habits.

Homeopathic Remedies

Arsenicum
Burning pain in pit of stomach quite soon after food, relieved by warm liquids. Sensation of weight like a stone in the stomach.

Bryonia
Discomfort in pit of stomach soon after food, "like a stone"; belching with acid liquid

(waterbrash) in back of throat; heartburn and dull pain in upper right abdomen not relieved by warm liquids (contrast *Arsenicum*).

Carbo Veg

Pain and tenderness in pit of stomach one-half hour after food. Abdomen feels heavy with waterbrash, bloating, offensive gas (which gives relief). The simplest food disagrees.

Chamomilla

(See also Abdominal Pain). Gas with abdominal cramping coming on after anger; red cheeks and perspiration. Bitter taste in mouth; pain in abdomen; worse by warmth.

Colocynthis

(See also Abdominal Pain). Bitter taste; abdomen distended; pain in abdomen; better by warmth.

Ignatia

(See also Abdominal Pain). Sour belching; much flatulence (passing gas) with rumbling in bowels; hiccough. "All gone" feeling and sinking in stomach made better by deep inspiration. Longs for indigestible foods. Often comes on after fright.

Ipecac

(See also Abdominal Pain). Nausea and vomiting; hiccough; gas; clean tongue; much saliva. Often comes on after eating indigestible foods, cakes, raisins.

Nux Vomica

Heartburn and gas from over-indulgence in coffee, tobacco, alcohol. Distended abdomen, bloated a few hours after eating. Worse in morning; waterbrash; ineffectual urge to vomit.

Pulsatilla

Bloating with a sensation of having eaten too much or a stone in the stomach one or two hours after food, especially after fats, warm food or drink. Regurgitates food and burps taste of food. Odd cravings for indigestible things or some special food or drink. Thirstless.

XXVI. INFLAMMATION (See Abscesses & Inflammation)

XXVII. INJURIES

There are many varieties of injuries to the body. Some are intentional such as tooth extractions and surgical operations; but most are unintentional cuts, scratches, bruises, sprains and strains, burns, bites and stings. Homeopathic remedies can greatly aid the injured person in his recovery. The first order of business is a thorough assessment of the injury. Any injury may have superficial manifestations but also deeper damage to tendons, nerves, blood vessels, bones and organs. If you are uncertain of the extent of injuries, it is best to consult a physician.

After rapid assessment, bleeding should be controlled. In general, this may be done by applying direct pressure to the site of the injury with a clean, moist cloth. Occasionally, bleeding is so profuse that other measures such as applying pressure to an artery may be required. For further training, a Red Cross First Aid course should be taken.

For control of pain and swelling, a cold, moist application is useful. Avoid placing ice directly against the skin.

To help bring the mind away from focusing on the pain, techniques of yoga breath awareness or childbirth breathing may be used.

In transporting injured patients, be cautious not to aggravate the injury. Consult a Red Cross First Aid Manual or take a First Aid course to learn how to transport injured patients.

This section is divided into five common categories of injury:

A. Wounds   (incised wounds, lacerated wounds, scratches and abrasions)
B. Bites, stings and puncture wounds
C. Bruises

D. Burns

E. Sprains and Strains

A. WOUNDS

Incised Wounds

Skin is cut by a sharp instrument which may have divided not only the skin but also more important structures underneath. Such a wound may require a physician's attention to repair it, particularly if it is a wide, gaping cut or involves deeper structures. This is especially true of wounds of the hands and feet. Careful inspection of even superficial wounds of these parts of the body is important to prevent loss of function.

If the cut involves only skin and no deeper structures are involved, the injured part should be soaked with **Calendula** lotion after thorough cleansing with water (soapy water if the edges are dirty). Then a dressing of **Calendula** ointment can be applied to protect the injury site. This process of soaking and dressing should be done daily until new skin has healed over (more often if the dressing becomes contaminated).

Hypericum ointment or lotion may be used alone or with **Calendula**. Some homeopaths feel that this remedy is more useful in wounds that have unusual pain associated with them. For both **Calendula** and **Hypericum** lotions, 1 teaspoon of the mother tincture is mixed in 1 pint of water.

Lacerated Wounds

This type of wound is usually the result of a blow by a blunt object. Not only is skin broken, but underlying tissue is damaged from the force of the blow. Frequently, the wound has been contaminated by dirt and foreign debris. **Arnica** should be given for the immediate injury and the wound cleansed and soaked well and covered with **Hypericum** or **Calendula** dressing. If the wound involves an area rich in nerves (e.g., finger tips), then **Hypericum** should be given in addition to **Arnica**, particularly if the pain shoots centrally.

Scratches and Abrasions

These are superficial but frequently very painful and potentially disfiguring injuries. Here, the top layer of skin is rubbed off and often dirt and tar ingrained in the raw skin. Cleansing with cold water of **Calendula** lotion will help, but in cases where foreign material has been ingrained, a physician should be seen for the necessary treatment to prevent dirt tattoo. After cleansing, the abrasion can be covered with **Calendula** ointment or lotion and/or **Hypericum** if there is pain.

B. BITES, STINGS AND PUNCTURE WOUNDS

Usually, these are of minor significance; but occasionally the wounds can become infected (human or animal bite); a person may be allergically hypersensitive to the toxin (bee or wasp sting); or a poison may be introduced (snake). Wounds which appear as lacerations should be treated as above.

For snake, severe animal bite or rabid dog bite, contact physician or emergency room immediately. Before the doctor is seen, however, **Hypericum** can help, especially if there is pain. For snake bite, **Ledum** is indicated.

For simple bee and wasp stings, mosquito bites and other puncture wounds:

Homeopathic Remedies

Apis

Bites that cause stinging pains and swelling or puffiness of any body part, particularly the eyes, ankles or hands.

Arnica

Helps alleviate soreness of affected area after bites. Can be used for bee and wasp stings that feel as though they are bruised.

Calendula

Lotion or ointment—useful externally

to help alleviate pain and decrease risk of infection.

Cantharis
Used after puncture by nettle or when pain is burning.

Hypericum
For internal use after horsefly bites, or when pains travel up the arm, or when fingertips are involved.

Ledum
Most used remedy in stings and mosquito bites. A few doses will help alleviate pain, swelling and counteract the effects of poison. Particularly useful when extremities are cold; after puncture by sharp instrument or after injections and shots where area is sore.

C. BRUISES

Bruises are the result of injuries from a blow by a blunt instrument to soft parts of the body, leading to swelling, discoloration and pain. Overexertion also can cause a sensation of being bruised.

Homeopathic Remedies

Arnica
Useful when muscles or soft tissues are
black and blue or are sore from overuse.
Should be given first in any injury.

Arnica Ointment
Used if muscle or soft tissue is bruised;
should *not* be used if skin is broken.

Calendula Ointment
Useful if bruise is associated with broken
skin.

Hypericum
Especially indicated if injuries or blows
occur to fingers, toes or spine, particularly
to the tailbone (coccyx).

Ledum
For blows to eye causing pain, swelling or
discoloration (black eye).   Useful after
injuries that *Arnica* fails to heal; or if parts
affected are cold.

Ruta
Helps alleviate pain and tenderness when
bruise occurs on bone (chin, elbow, skull)
and   pain   is   felt   on   surface   of   bone,

particularly in places where tendons attach to the bone.

D. BURNS

Three degrees of burns are:
First Degree: Redness and pain; sunburn.
Second Degree: Has blisters.
Third Degree: Severe, deep burns of all layers of skin and below.

Immediately remove the patient from the cause of the burn; remove the affected part from heat or wash off chemical irritant with copious amounts of cool or lukewarm water. Do not scrub the affected parts as skin and underlying flesh may tear away. Immediately cool the area with cool water, *not ice.*

In very serious burns involving large areas of the body, there are two immediate dangers: one is fluid loss into the space as the tissues swell. Keep the patient hydrated if he can tolerate drinking. The second is the swelling itself which may cause problems.   If the leg swells, for example, the swelling may cut off circulation to the extremity.

Biochemics

Kali Mur

For first and second degree burns with redness and blisters; especially if there is white or greyish exudate over the wound.

Homeopathic Remedies

Arnica

Should be given at once. The two-hundredth potency is preferred, but the thirtieth potency will do and may be repeated several times, 2 to 6 hours apart. After the initial dose of *Arnica*, follow with a dose of **Cantharis** to relieve pain. Repeat every ten minutes until relief is obtained. Whenever pain returns, **Cantharis** should be given again.

Hypericum

Hypericum lotion should be applied externally, particularly in first degree burns. In cases of electrical burns, the skin manifestations may be very deceiving. Extensive tissue damage may occur beneath the surface of the skin without showing much skin destruction. **Cantharis** should be given immediately, and immediate medical attention should be sought.

E. SPRAINS AND STRAINS

These injuries are the result of stretching either the muscles or the ligaments too vigorously. Take **Arnica** internally as soon as possible after the injury and apply ice packs externally to area (use

a moist rather than a dry application) to keep
down the swelling and help control the pain.
Several homeopathic remedies are indicated after
the initial *Arnica*, depending on how the symptoms
develop.

Homeopathic Remedies

Bryonia

Joint becomes painful and swollen, distended with fluid. Particularly indicated
when joint is painful on the least amount
of movement.

Rhus Tox

Indicated for hot, swollen, painful joints.
Pain generally is of tearing character; feels
better with warm application. Initially,
movement is painful, but the pain gets
better with motion (in contrast to *Bryonia*).
Gentle rubbing makes the pain better.

Ruta

Pain feels closer to the bone and can be
associated with hard swelling where the
tendon is attached to the bone. Pain is
aching in character and is made worse by
every movement of the injured part. (For
example, each time the muscle is stretched,
the injured tendon will hurt.) Patient

restless, but not to the degree of *Rhus Tox.*

XXVIII. MEASLES

This is a highly infectious illness of childhood that usually occurs 9 to 14 days after being exposed to another child with measles. It begins with high fever and lassitude and is followed by a harsh, barking cough, inflammation of the eyes and runny nose. The rash begins three days later, seen first on the face.

In the early stages, if measles is suspected, **Aconite, Belladonna** or **Ferrum Phos** should be given if their symptoms are present (see Fever). Other remedies are:

Homeopathic Remedies

Apis
High temperature; very hot; wanting covers off; eyes sore; irritable and tearful. Pains stinging in quality.

Bryonia
Chest involved with tiresome, dry, painful cough. Headache with dry mouth and intense thirst for cold water. Generally, the rash appears late and the disease runs a regular course. Person lies motionless.

Gelsemium
Fever is a prominent symptom; very high

temperature; sluggishness, apathy. There is a watery nasal discharge which excoriates the nose and upper lip. Harsh, barking, croupy cough; may have hoarseness. Eyelids droopy and heavy. Should be continued after rash, particularly if it is red and itchy. Can have headache at the base of skull.

Pulsatilla

Generally indicated later in the illness when fever has subsided or entirely disappeared. Often has runny nose and eyes with yellow, milky discharge. Troublesome cough and wants to sit up to cough. Child cries easily and wants to be comforted.

XXIX. MUMPS

A common childhood infection; one-third of cases have no symptoms. In cases where symptoms are present, the patient can have high fever or headache and swelling of cheeks and glands under the ear. Usually occurs two or three weeks after exposure to a case.

Biochemics

Ferrum Phos

Indicated in initial fever stage.

Kali Mur
Indicated when there is swelling, particularly when pain on swallowing is present.

Homeopathic Remedies

Belladonna
This is the most important homeopathic remedy for mumps and is associated with its typical fever symptoms; throbbing, burning skin, especially on the face, without relief from sweating, and nervous irritability. Glands are swollen, hot and red, very sensitive to pressure and often worse on the right side; pains may extend to the ear. This remedy is also indicated when the swelling suddenly subsides and is followed by a throbbing headache and delirium.

Pulsatilla
Used when there is involvement of the testicles and mammary glands. Thick coating on the tongue; mouth is dry and patient is without thirst, even with the fever. The patient tends to be weepy and demands constant attention.

Rhus Tox
Mood is sad (see also *Pulsatilla*) and there is extreme restlessness with constant desire to change position. Glands under ears are swollen,

worse on left side; cheekbones sensitive to touch; jaws crack when chewing. Pains in other joints relieved by limbering up.

XXX. NAUSEA AND VOMITING

Although nausea and vomiting can be symptoms of chronic, deep-seated illnesses, more often they are transient, coming on quickly after a particular inciting stimulus. The 24 or 48 hour "flu" will commonly occur at one time or another in most families. Moreover, food poisoning (called ptomaine poisoning) comes after eating spoiled food (usually after catered affairs, picnics and dining out). In general, sips of hot water are comforting, as are warm applications to the abdomen. In addition to the nausea and vomiting, the person sometimes has diarrhea. In such a case, give a remedy that fits the whole picture rather than being distracted by two apparently different conditions.

Homeopathic Remedies

Arsenicum
Useful for the bad effects of spoiled food, drinking ice-cold water, or eating ice cream. Characteristic prostration, restlessness and burning pain; nausea with retching; extreme irritation of the stomach, frequently associated with diarrhea. Temporary relief from warm drinks.

Bryonia

Usually from overeating; violent pain in abdomen with severe vomiting; thirsty but water returns as soon as it reaches the stomach. Nausea and vomiting come on as soon as patient sits up; better lying down, perfectly still with limbs flexed. Bitter eructations, with nauseating taste.

Chamomilla

Much vomiting; belches smell like rotten eggs; violent retching; bitter vomiting; makes violent efforts to vomit as if stomach would tear. Nausea after coffee.

Colocynthis

Vomiting and diarrhea frequently accompanying colicky pain; pain relieved by pressure and bending double. Pain predominates the picture and should guide the prescriber (see also Abdominal Pain).

Ipecac

Persistent nausea and vomiting; vomiting preceded by much nausea; nausea not relieved by vomiting; often comes after eating rich foods, pastry, pork, and foods that are difficult to digest. Tongue usually clear or only slightly coated. Can be accompanied by diarrhea.

Nux Vomica

Sour taste and nausea in the morning after eating. *Nux* patient generally has overindulged in food, mental work and sex. Nausea and vomiting with much retching. Difficult to vomit. Sensation of a stone in the stomach an hour after eating.

Pulsatilla

Like *Nux Vomica*, the *Pulsatilla* patient who vomits also suffers from a generalized indigestion (see section on indigestion). Vomiting of food taken long before; mood is weepy.

XXXI. PAIN

Pain should not be feared, but appreciated. It is the body telling you that something is wrong; thus it serves a protective function. It is not only a warning guide but also aids the physician in making a more precise diagnosis. It is wise not to suppress or dull pain without first correcting the cause because even if the actual painful stimulus is removed, the underlying causal factor may be worsening. Drugs such as aspirin, acetaminophen and stronger drugs are thus discouraged. Indiscriminate use of pain killers leads to suppression of vitally needed symptoms and also can easily become habit-forming or have unpleasant side effects.

Pain indicates that something in the body is wrong. Its location, type, intensity and character should be analyzed and used as a guide to the correct remedy. Homeopathic prescription will help alleviate pain by getting at the root cause.

Recurrent pain should be a stimulus to re-examine habits, feelings and modes of expression which may be the cause of the pain.

XXXII. POISON IVY OR POISON OAK

Reactions to these irritants vary from mild itching to severe, systemic problems such as difficulty breathing. In general, the biochemics can be used as indicated for inflammatory processes. The most useful homeopathic remedy is **Rhus Tox**. Be careful not to contact unexposed areas with those areas where eruption is present. This will spread the irritation and rash. Relief is possible from wet applications (most often warm). The use of topical ointments and lotions should be avoided.

XXXIII. POISONING

In any case of suspected poisoning, take the person to the nearest emergency room or call the local poison control center. This center will give you the appropriate first aid instructions. In addition, it is important to find the container so that proper identification and treatment can be made.

XXXIV. RESPIRATORY INFECTION

When the lining of the respiratory tract (nose, throat, windpipe and lungs) becomes inflamed, it is a sign that a person is attempting to regain his inner balance. It may also involve eyes, ears and occasionally other body systems such as muscles and joints. There are general symptoms such as emotional changes, change in energy level, fevers, chills, etc. Localized signs and symptoms are also found, such as discharges from nose, throat, eyes and ears, etc. The two primary symptoms of respiratory infection are cough and sore throat. What follows are sections on cough and sore throat. In addition to the treatment suggested in these sections, one should avoid mucus producing foods such as dairy products, meat, sweets and grains. Instead, one should eat vegetable broths, fresh juices, tea and fresh fruits. (See Fever.)

A. COUGHS AND COLDS

Coughing usually results from irritation of the air passages. An upper respiratory virus, smoking or environmental pollution often initiate the process. Cough is generally a beneficial phenomenon, enabling the lining of the respiratory system to remove the offending agent by forceful expulsion.

Coughing should not be suppressed by cough medicines, narcotics or sprays since this may drive the illness deeper into the system, cover up important symptoms needed by the doctor for correct homeopathic prescribing, and tend to worsen the infection since the material causing irritation cannot be removed by the cough.

Acute coughs, especially those associated with "colds" and sore throats, can be helped by homeopathic home prescribing. More chronic coughs should be evaluated by a qualified homeopathic physician.

Biochemics

Ferrum Phos

Indicated in the first stages of an upper respiratory infection with cough where there is fever.

Kali Mur

Indicated if there is a white coating on the tongue. Also indicated if the discharge from the nose or back of the throat is white. Swelling is a major indication—whether it be stuffiness and nasal congestion, closing off the ear canal with resultant fluid buildup in the ear, or swollen tonsils and glands.

Homeopathic Remedies

Aconite

To be given at the first sign of respiratory infection, especially if it comes on after exposure to a dry, cold draft. Frequent sneezing, fever, thirst and restlessness at night. Cough is dry, with a hard ringing sound. Generally only useful during the onset of the infection.

Arsenicum

The hallmark of this remedy is burning pains relieved by heat. Discharges from the nose are thin, watery and burn the skin underneath the nose. There is thirst for small amounts of water. Patient is irritable and restless. Cough is worse lying down and feels suffocating, can resemble wheezing of asthma and is generally dry and associated with burning of the chest. Usually worse at night after awakening the patient.

Belladonna

Patient has red, hot face without relief from perspiration. Violent onset after exposure to chilling, particularly by the head. Dryness is a hallmark of the remedy except for perspiration on covered parts of the body. Cough is dry, tickling and comes in violent paroxysms. When the patient coughs, his head feels as if it will burst. Coughing fits will often end in sneezing or a whoop. The child frequently will cry before the coughing fit begins.

Bryonia

The person requiring this remedy is inclined to lie perfectly still, objecting strongly to being moved and, in fact, will even object to people being in the same room with him. Wants to be left alone. Symptoms are worse with least movement. Patient is thirsty for large amounts of cold liquids, although hot drinks may actually help the cough. The infection has a tendency to travel downward into the chest. Coughing is associated with pain and is hard, dry and spasmodic, shaking the whole body, and associated with soreness in the chest as well as a "bursting" headache. In such a patient, illness is slow to develop. Nasal discharge is watery; lips and mouth are dry; expectoration, if present, is difficult. Patient feels faint on rising. Cough is aggravated from coming into warm room from cold air.

Carbo Veg

Indicated in the bronchitis of old people with profuse yellow, foul-smelling expectoration associated with difficulty in breathing. Much rattling in the chest and a sensation of burning. Cough begins with itching in larynx and is spasmodic in nature with gagging and some occasional vomiting of mucus. Generally associated with chills and thirst; occasional exhausting sweats.

Dulcamara

Cold usually follows exposure to cold, wet weather or becoming chilled when overheated. Sneezing severe and eyes and nose are generally streaming, although nose alternates being stuffy in cold and runny in warmth, with either clear or yellow discharge.

Gelsemium

Patient feels very sluggish. Infection usually comes on after exposure to warm, humid weather. Patient has chills, particularly along the spine and feels alternately hot and cold. Often associated with headache and heavy feeling in the eyelids and limbs. Cough is dry and tearing, associated with a sore chest. As with *Bryonia*, the patient desires to be left alone. Patient has much sneezing, with a feeling of dryness in the nose in spite of an excoriating discharge and can have a bad taste in the mouth and a thick, yellowish, coated tongue.

Hepar Sulph

Indicated in infections which spread from throat to ears. Discharge at first is watery and then becomes thick, yellow and offensive, with nose becoming swollen and painful. Desire to be well covered and can be feverish and hypersensitive. Cough (if there is one) is husky and hoarse with a loose edge which frequently leads to a fit of choking. The infection usually follows exposure to cold, dry weather. Stitches in the throat tend to extend to the ear on swallowing.

Merc Sol

Cough with yellow, pussy expectoration, made worse from lying on the

right side; at night; in a warm bed.
Much sneezing, nostrils raw with
yellow-green nasal discharge that smells
bad.

Nux Vomica

Infection starts from exposure to dry
coldness or after overindulgence of
food or sex, and is associated with
much sneezing with the nose alternately blocked or running. Generally stopped up at night and streaming in a
warm room and during the daytime.
Feels extremely chilly and can't get
warm. Will shudder after drinking
fluids or from the least movement.
Alternate chills and fever; excessively
irritable. Cough is short, dry and
fatiguing, accompanied by headache
and soreness in abdominal area.

Pulsatilla

Thirstless and peevish; constantly
wanting attention or to be held. Infection is associated with thick, yellow,
bland discharge in throat and eyes
which is worse in the morning. Patient
has chills up and down the back. Fever
present. Used in later stages of respiratory infection.

Rhus Tox

Cough worse from midnight to morning, during a chill, or when putting hands out of bed. Usually associated with influenza with aching bones; bronchial coughs of old people with expectoration of small plugs of mucus.

Spongia

Used in coughs associated with dryness of the air passages, burning of the larynx which is sensitive to touch. Cough is better after eating or drinking, especially warm drinks. Can be associated with asthma where wheezing is worse in cold air.

Sticta

Cough is associated with head colds, sneezing and runny nose. Cough is dry and hacking and worse in the evening and during inspiration.

B. SORE THROAT

This is a common ailment in children under twelve, although adults also can have it. At this young age, the child cannot always describe the details of the pain. To be a successful prescriber, learn to be a careful observer. In anyone, a sore throat must be treated with respect for it may herald a more serious systemic illness. If prone to sore throats, consult a homeopathic physician for constitutional treatment. In the meantime, keeping the neck covered with a scarf will help to prevent recurrent infections. Gargling with warm salt water helps to reduce the pain. The following remedies, if given promptly, will speed the recovery.

Biochemics

Ferrum Phos
Throat dry, red, inflamed, with much pain (frequent doses needed). Throat burning with pain. Associated with fever.

Kali Mur
When swelling of the glands and tonsils sets in, give *Kali Mur* and *Ferrum Phos* in alternation. Throat ulcerated with white or grayish patches. Tongue coated white.

Homeopathic Remedies

Aconite
Should be used in first stage of a sore

throat which comes on violently, especially after being exposed to dry, cold wind. Burning, dry, very red throat. Fever, and hurts to swallow.

Apis
Stinging. Pains in throat, which is swollen; absence of thirst; worse with warm drinks.

Arsenicum
Burning pains in throat relieved by hot drinks; although patient is thirsty, sips only small amounts of liquids.

Belladonna
Throat is dry and burns like fire. Tonsils inflamed and bright red. Tongue bright red or looks like a strawberry. Averse to liquids because of pain. Face red, hot, with dilated pupils. Patient's mood is restless, agitated, sometimes delirious.

Bryonia
Dryness, scraped, constricted feeling is worse coming into warm room; lips dry; tongue coated white. Desire to be motionless and left alone.

Cantharis

Burning in mouth, pharynx and throat. Blisters in mouth and on tongue. Great difficulty swallowing liquids. Throat feels like fire.

Gelsemium

The sore throat develops slowly over several days, often with exposure in warm, moist, relaxing weather. Sluggishness is the hallmark of this remedy. Tonsils swollen and throat feels rough and burning. Swallowing causes pain in throat and ear. May have pain in neck muscles extending up to an area just behind the angle of the jaw near the ears. Usually no thirst. Chills up and down the back.

Hepar Sulph

Sore throat with well-established "cold." When swallowing, there is a sensation of a splinter or fishbone caught in the throat, or a sensation of a lump in the throat. Pain on swallowing shooting from throat to ear. Very irritable and sensitive to the least draft.

Ignatia

Feeling of lump stuck in throat. Suits

particularly the over-dramatic patient.

Mercurius Sol
Raw, smarting throat. Foul breath. Thirst despite moist mouth and much salivation. Thick, yellow coating on tongue. Painful swallowing but must swallow because of increased saliva.

Nux Vomica
Rough, scraped feeling. Tickling after waking in morning. Often comes on after overeating the night before. Pain shoots into ears.

XXXV. SKIN DISEASES
These are generally manifestations of chronic disease and should be treated as such by a physician.

XXXVI. SPRAINS AND STRAINS (See Injuries)

XXXVII. STINGS (See Injuries)

XXXVIII. STYES

Styes are infections of the glands lining the eyelids, resulting in small pustules embedded in the eyelids. Generally, warm, moist applications are useful in either bringing the stye to a head or in assisting drainage once the stye has come to a head. These should be applied several times a day for twenty minutes or so.

As in any inflammatory condition, the biochemics may be used as well as additional homeopathic remedies.

Biochemics

Calcarea Sulph
Always "after the pus has found a vent." To follow *Silicea* to complete the drainage.

Ferrum Phos
For the initial signs of inflammation where there is redness of the eyelid margin but no swelling.

Kali Mur
When swelling of the lid has begun.

Silicea
To help swelling form a head. Continue dosage until stye drains.

Homeopathic Remedies

Apis
Styes with sudden, piercing, stinging pains are typical of *Apis*. Eyelids swollen, red.

Pulsatilla
Eyelids inflamed; often stick together;

discharge creamy and yellowish. Styes especially on upper lid. Most important is typical temperament and modalities of weeping, peevishness and changeable moods.

XXXIX. TEETHING (See Dentition)

XL. TOOTHACHE

Dental hygiene is of upmost importance in overall health. Diet is perhaps the best and most important aspect in the prevention of tooth decay. Refrain from use of refined sugars and grains, artificial colorings and flavorings. Fresh green vegetables (raw and cooked), whole grains, beans, fresh fruit and dairy products are indispensable. Brushing, gentle dental flossing, and gum massage with a clean forefinger are also important, as are regular checkups with a dentist.

Biochemics

Ferrum Phos
Swollen cheeks or signs of systemic infection such as fever.

Kali Mur
If there is swelling.

Magnesia Phos
Intense, shooting pain that is relieved with

pressure or hot liquids. Pain is increased by slightest movement and is worse with cold liquids.

Homeopathic Remedies

Arnica
Useful before and after tooth extraction and dental work, or after injury to the teeth.

Arsenicum
Teeth feel sore and long; burning pain; worse after midnight; relieved by warmth.

Belladonna
Throbbing pains in teeth associated with dry, hot face and restlessness.

Mercurius Sol
Teeth tender and aching; worse from cold drinks and foods, from chewing; at night and from warmth of the bed. Metallic taste; foul breath; swelling around the jaw.

Pulsatilla
Toothache relieved by holding cold water in the mouth; worse from warm drinks; dry mouth without thirst. Peevish, desires comfort.

XLI. TRAVEL SICKNESS

Homeopathic Remedies

Ignatia
Indicated if there is nausea associated with a feeling of trembling and fright.

Nux Vomica
A horrible, queezy nausea, which may be associated with a headache, usually felt at the back of the head or over one eye. Bloated feeling; much gagging and retching which can produce vomitus. Patient seeks to be warm.

Rhus Tox
Especially valuable in air sickness. Patient feels faint on attempting to rise. Complete loss of appetite. Can have severe frontal headache. Scalp sensitive to touch. Patient has unquenchable thirst, with dry mouth and throat.

XLII. WOUNDS (See Injuries)

Section C

MATERIA MEDICA

Materia Medica

Biochemics

I. CALCAREA PHOSPHORICA
(Calcarea Phos)

Generalities

Complaints during teething, such as diarrhea, colic, fever.

Uses

1. Dentition
2. Toothache

II. CALCAREA SULPHURICA
(Calcarea Sulph)

Generalities

Presence of draining pus is general indication; useful in cases of boils, carbuncles, abscesses and pus-forming inflammation when matter is discharging or continuing to ooze.

Uses

1. Abscess
2. Styes

III. FERRUM PHOSPHORICUM
(Ferrum Phos)

Generalities

Indicated in ailments of generalized inflammation, characterized by pain, fever, redness, inflammation of multiple sites, quickened pulse. Used for fevers and inflammation before pus accumulates.

Modalities

Worse:	Motion
Better:	Cold and applications

Clinical Picture

Head:	Aching with rush of blood; headache from heat of sun.
Eyes:	Red, burning, sore; sensation of grain of sand under lid.
Ears:	First stage of earache, with tension, throbbing and heat.
Nose:	Bleeding, especially in children.
Face:	Flushed.
Tongue:	Clean and reddened.
Throat:	Sore, dry, red, inflamed, painful; no pus yet.
Respiratory:	First stages of cough.

Skin: Measles and fever of scarlet fever
                 (first stage); bleeding in general.

Dosage

Not to be used past dark since it may cause
sleeplessness.

Uses

1. Abdominal pain
2. Abscesses
3. Bleeding
4. Chicken Pox
5. Ear problems
6. Fever
7. Headache
8. Hemorrhoids
9. Hoarseness
10. Measles
11. Mumps
12. Respiratory Infection
    a. Cough and cold
    b. Sore throat
13. Styes
14. Toothache

IV. KALI MURIATICUM
(Kali Mur)

Generalities

Useful in patients with white bodily discharges. Corresponds generally to the second stage of inflammation when fluid is accumulating and pus is beginning to form. For the Home Prescriber, *Kali Mur* is very useful in ear problems; ears feel full, decrease in hearing due to swelling. Often there are snapping, cracking sounds on blowing the nose or swallowing.

Clinical Picture

Ears: Deafness or earache from congestion and swelling of middle ear or Eustachian tubes.
Nose: White, thick discharge.
Tongue: Gray-white, coated (a very important indication for the prescriber).
Throat: Whitish-gray; spots on enlarged tonsils; pain on swallowing; cough.

Uses

1. Abscesses
2. Asthma
3. Bleeding

4. Chicken Pox
5. Ear problems
6. Fever
7. Hayfever
8. Injury
    a. Burns
9. Mumps
10. Respiratory infection
    a. Coughs and colds
    b. Sore throat
11. Styes
12. Toothache

V. MAGNESIA PHOSPHORICA
(Magnesia Phos)

Generalities

Chiefly a "pain" remedy. Indicated in ailments of contracted, spasmodic, cramping, boring, constrictive pains; changing locality of pains. Especially useful in abdominal or menstrual cramps and minor back spasms.

Modalities
Worse: Cold; light; touch; night.
Better: Bending over; external warmth; pressure.

Clinical Picture
Head: Pains shooting, shifting, spasmodic; better by external warmth.
Face: Spasmodic pain.
Tongue: Clean.
Teeth: Toothache, shooting pains relieved by warmth.
Abdomen: Pain with gas, forcing patient to double over. Better with rubbing, warmth, belching, drawing legs up.
Back and   Aching, boring, darting pains any-
Extremities: where.

Dosage
Works best when twenty grains can be dissolved in a quarter glass of warm water and sipped slowly every fifteen minutes.

Uses
1. Abdominal pain
2. Asthma
3. Hayfever
4. Headache
5. Hiccough
6. Toothache

VI. NATRUM PHOSPHORICUM
(Natrum Phos)

Generalities

People who need this biochemic often suffer from stomach troubles and abnormal bowel habits; diarrhea (often with greenish tinge and sour-smelling) or constipation. Gas and bloating in abdomen which cannot be relieved by passing gas. Sour risings from stomach to throat. Discharges from various parts of body are in general a golden-yellow color.

Clinical Picture

Mouth: Golden-yellow coating on tongue, throat and roof of mouth.

Stomach: Abdominal pain, especially in children with signs of acidity. Gas.

Uses
1. Abdominal pain

VII. NATRUM SULPHURICUM
(Natrum Sulph)

Generalities

Called the "washerman" of the biochemics because it removes excess water from the system. Useful in problems associated with rainy weather; patient feels changes from dry to wet weather; cannot even tolerate foods or plants taken from water (fish). Useful in swelling. In high homeopathic potency, it is useful in treatment of chronic problems, but as a biochemic in Home Prescribing, it is best suited for asthma and fluid retention.

Modalities

Worse: Damp weather; damp basements.
Better: Dry weather; pressure; changing position

Clinical Picture

Tongue: May have brownish, thick coating.
Respiratory: Asthma brought on in, or made worse by damp weather; often a-wakens patient at 4:00 or 5:00 a.m. Rattling in chest with thick expectoration.
Extremities: Swelling from fluid retention in ankles, feet, hands, etc. "Rheumatism" with aching or stiffness of joints made worse by dampness.

Uses

1. Asthma

VIII. SILICEA

Generalities

Use cautiously. Ripens abscesses; promotes drainage of pus. Once pus appears and no new material is found in the boil or abscess, follow with *Calcarea Sulph*, which promotes healing while pus is draining.

Uses

1. Abscesses
2. Styes

Homeopathic Remedies

I. ACONITUM NAPELLUS
(Aconite) (Monkshood)

Generalities

The remedy is given at first signs of colds or sore throats, especially those coming on suddenly after exposure to cold winds or drafts. Illness comes on suddenly, with great violence. Discharges are profuse. Most predominant general symptom in *Aconite* case is fear and anxious restlessness. Very sensitive to pain. May have painful inflammation without pus formation. Patients requiring this remedy tend to be strong and robust rather than sickly.

Modalities
Worse: In evening and night; violent emotions; lying on affected side.
Better: In open air, warmth, rest.

Clinical Picture
Mind: Great fear, anxiety, restlessness.
Head: Heavy, hot, bursting, pulsating sensation, worse on rising.
Face: Red hot, flushed; becomes pale on rising.

Eyes:	Feel dry and hot; lids swollen.
Throat:	Red, dry and constricted. Intense thirst.
Lungs:	Shortness of breath; hoarse, dry, croupy cough.
Heart:	Pulse full, hard, tense and bounding.
Skin:	Red hot, dry, burning.

Uses

1. Bleeding
2. Collapse or Shock
3. Croup
4. Diarrhea
5. Ear problems
6. Eye disorders
7. Fever
8. Headache
9. Hoarseness
10. Measles
11. Respiratory infection
    a. Coughs and colds
    b. Sore throat

II. APIS MELLIFICA
(Apis) (Honey Bee)

Generalities
Burning, sharp, stinging pains with redness and swelling (like bee sting); swelling both sudden and chronic, general and local in any tissue; especially prominent in the ankles, mouth, throat, eyelids, and around the eyes; absence of thirst. Very tender or sensitive to touch, as if bruised.

Modalities
Worse: With warmth, pressure; afternoon; lying down; wet.

Better: By cold (room, air or applications).

Clinical Picture
Eyes: Lids swollen, red, burning and stinging.

Mouth: Red, shiny, puffy.

Stomach: Thirstless, craving for milk.

Abdomen: Extremely tender, sore, bruised on pressure.

Skin: Swelling with bites.

Uses
1. Abscesses
2. Headache

3. Injuries
   a. Bites, stings, puncture wounds
4. Measles
5. Respiratory infections
   a. Sore throat
6. Styes

III. ARNICA MONTANA
(Arnica) (Leopard's Bane)

Generalities
Always the first remedy used internally for injury or overexertion. Patient has feeling of bruised soreness with aching and pressing pains; hyperacuteness of senses; fear of being approached or touched. Should be used externally over bruised area *only if there is no broken skin.* Otherwise, infection will result.

Modalities
Worse: Evenings and night; touch, pressure, physical exertion.

Better: Open air; lying down; with heat.

Clinical Picture
Mind: Fears touch or approach; feels bruised.

Head: Hot, with cold body.

Throat: Hoarseness from overuse of voice.

Skin: Black and blue; bruises.

Extremities: Cannot walk or raise arms due to soreness.

Uses
1. Abscesses
2. Bleeding
3. Collapse and Shock

4. Eye disorders
5. Headache
6. Hoarseness
7. Injury
   a. Wounds
   b. Lacerations
   c. Bruises
   d. Bites, stings, puncture wounds
   e. Burns
   f. Sprains and Strains
8. Toothache

IV. ARSENICUM ALBUM
(Arsenicum) (Arsenic Trioxide)

Generalities
Characterized by burning pains, relieved by heat; anxious, restless, weak and chilly with an air of fear and hopelessness. Tries to find relief in motion; always moving. Feels cold. Complains of general weakness which is out of proportion to the apparent cause. Discharges are excoriating (burn the skin). Strong, intense thirst; drinks often but little at a time; cold water disagrees.

Modalities
Worse: Cold air; after midnight (particularly from 1:00 to 3:00 a.m.).

Better: Warmth, open air; relieved by sweat.

Clinical Picture
Mind: Great anguish and restlessness.

Nose: Thin, watery discharge that burns the skin around nose.

Throat: Burning pain, relieved by hot drinks.

Stomach: Aversion to sight or smell of food; burning pain.

Stool: Diarrhea, with burning of rectum.

Lungs: Unable to lie down; fears suffocation; cough worse after midnight.

Extremities: Trembling, twitching.

Uses

1. Asthma
2. Bleeding
3. Diarrhea
4. Hayfever
5. Indigestion
6. Nausea and vomiting
7. Respiratory infection
   a. Coughs and colds
   b. Sore throat
8. Toothache

V. BELLADONNA
(Deadly Nightshade)

Generalities

Characterized by sudden, violent onset and rapid progression of symptoms. High temperature; congestion; redness and throbbing with sweat only on covered parts. Predominantly right-sided; hypersensitivity to all sensation with heightened nervous excitability that can cause acute delirium; twitching of muscles and spasms of internal organs with sensations of constriction or fullness. Pains are usually throbbing and stabbing; appear suddenly and then disappear and reappear again.

Modalities

Worse:	Touch or motion; cold, particularly drafts; lying down; 3:00 p.m. to midnight.
Better:	Heat; sitting still and upright; covering up.

Clinical Picture

Mind:	Acuteness of all senses; tends toward delirium; restless, especially while sleeping; may cry out during sleep because of nightmares.
Head:	Throbbing pain with sensation of fullness, especially in forehead.
Face:	Red, especially cheeks; hot; dry.

Eyes: Pupils dilated; eyes feel swollen; glassy-eyed.
Ears: Tearing pain.
Tongue: Red on edges; white with red spots, (strawberry looking).
Throat: Dry, red, constricted; painful swelling.
Stomach: No appetite; either extreme thirst or aversion to liquids.
Lungs: Tickling; short, dry cough; worse at night. Larynx very painful.
Skin: Dry, hot, "burns" your hand; glands swollen, tender; perspiration on covered parts.

Uses
1. Abdominal pain
2. Bleeding
3. Ear problems
4. Fever
5. Headache
6. Hoarseness
7. Measles
8. Mumps
9. Respiratory infection
    a. Coughs and colds
    b. Sore throat
10. Toothache

VI. BRYONIA ALBA
(Bryonia) (Wild Hops)

Generalities

Of all the remedies with aggravation from motion, *Bryonia* is the leader. This modality is the hallmark of *Bryonia*. Markedly affected by motion; the least change of position in some distant part aggravates the pain; great thirst for large quantities at long intervals. Typical *Bryonia* patient is irritable, inclined to be vehement; angry outbursts when disturbed; often has dark hair and complexion. All internal surfaces feel dry from mouth to joints, lungs, abdomen and pelvic area. Symptoms usually develop slowly (contrast with *Aconite, Belladonna*).

Modalities
Worse: Motion; inhalation; touch; sitting up; warmth.

Better: Lying on painful side; absolute rest; cold; eating cold things; firm pressure.

Clinical Picture
Mind: Irritable, doesn't want to be bothered; desires seclusion.

Head: Bursting, splitting headaches as if everything pressed out. Worse on motion.

Nose: Dry.
Mouth: Lips parched, dry, cracked; bitter taste.
Tongue: White coating.
Stomach: Nausea and faintness upon rising; vomiting of bile and water immediately after eating; warm drinks are vomited.
Abdomen: Sensitive to touch.
Stool: Constipated; stools dry, as if burnt.
Lungs: Dry, hacking cough, especially at night; must sit up when coughing.

Uses

1. Abdominal pain
2. Bleeding
3. Diarrhea
4. Fever
5. Headache
6. Indigestion
7. Injuries
   a. Sprains and strains
8. Measles
9. Nausea and vomiting
10. Respiratory infection
    a. Coughs and colds
    b. Sore throat

VII. CALENDULA OFFICINALIS
(Calendula) (Marigold)

Generalities

Injuries involving cutting, tearing or other mechanical forms of injury; damage to surface of skin, exposing underlying living tissue; use externally as ointment or lotion (mother tincture diluted with water); provides protection against infection; promotes healing.

Dosage and Administration

Always use externally. Lotion is prepared by diluting 1 teaspoon *Calendula* mother tincture to one cup water. Lotion is useful when short-term soaking is indicated; ointment should be used for longer applications (overnight).

Uses

1. Eye disorders
2. Hemorrhoids
3. Injuries
   a. Wounds
      i. Incised
      ii. Lacerated
   b. Bites, scratches, puncture wounds
   c. Bruises
   d. Burns

VIII. CANTHARIS VESICATORIA
(Cantharis) (Spanish Fly)

Generalities

Used for burns or scalds. Excessive burning pains (eyes, mouth, throat, stomach, intestinal tract); frequent urge to urinate with burning; passing a few drops of urine at a time; stringy, tenacious discharges from mucous membranes. Vesicles or blisters full of yellowish fluid quickly becoming filled with pus, burning like fire. Anxious restlessness ending in rage. Used for burns.

Modalities

Worse: Night; cold; pressure; coffee.
Better: Lying down.

Clinical Picture

Throat: Burning in mouth and throat; difficult to swallow liquids.

Stomach: Burning sensation of esophagus and stomach. Burning thirst, with aversion to all fluids.

Bladder: Intolerable urge to urinate.

Skin: Burns with blisters. Vesicles that burn and itch.

Uses

1. Injuries
   a. Bites, stings, puncture wounds
   b. Burns
2. Respiratory infection
   a. Sore throat

IX. CARBO VEGETABILIS
(Carbo Veg) (Vegetable Charcoal)

Generalities

Patient exhibits mental and physical sluggishness and symptoms come on slowly; generalized weakness of all functions, especially digestion; often fat, torpid, lazy. Complaints of coldness (general or local). Symptoms may date to inadequate recovery from previous exhausting disease. Pains usually described as burning, pressing pains. Must have fresh air; wishes to be fanned.

Modalities

Worse: Morning and evening; exertion; cold; tight clothes at abdomen.

Better: Passing gas; rest; being fanned.

Clinical Picture

Head: Aches from overindulgence.

Face: Puffy, gray-blue; pale.

Nose: Bleeds daily.

Stomach: Belching, heaviness, fullness and sleepiness. Contractive pain extending to chest, with distention of abdomen; distended with flatulent colic; simplest food disagrees. Aversion to milk, meats and fatty foods.

Respiratory: Wheezing in old people.
Skin: Blue; cold; moist.

Uses
1. Asthma
2. Bleeding
3. Collapse and shock
4. Hoarseness
5. Indigestion
6. Respiratory infection
   a. Coughs and colds

X. CHAMOMILLA
(German Chamomille)

Generalities
Chief symptoms are emotional, which usually lead to body disturbances. Frequently found in children who are restless, irritable, whining, and colicky. Sensitive, especially to pain. Thirsty, hot, numb sensation with unbearable pains. (Mental calmness, constipation rule against *Chamomilla*).

Modalities
Worse: Heat; anger; night; with wind.
Better: Being carried; warm, wet weather.

Clinical Picture
Ears: Feel hot; pain driving patient frantic. Child better being carried, pampered.
Teeth: Teething children who are cross and complaining; toothache after warm drinks.
Face: Hot with redness only on one side.
Tongue: Yellow coat.
Stomach: Acid, belching.
Abdomen: Colic, gas after anger. Red cheeks, hot perspiration.
Stool: Hot, green, watery; looks like chopped eggs and spinach.

Uses
1. Abdominal pain
2. Dentition
3. Diarrhea
4. Ear problems
5. Indigestion
6. Nausea and vomiting

XI. COLOCYNTHIS
(Bitter Cucumber)

Generalities
Ill effects of suppressed anger. Usually adopted for women with sedentary habits, often heavy. Severe, tearing pains relieved by pressure; cramping, pains especially in abdomen causing patient to double over. Often indicated in changing seasons, when air is cold but sun still heats the body.

Modalities
Worse: Suppressed emotion; least amount of food.

Better: Pressure; heat; bending over; escape of gas; passing stool.

Clinical Picture
Mind: Irritable when pains come.

Abdomen: Sensation of stones; abdomen feels like it will burst; bruised feeling; soreness around navel; worse with least amount of food.

Stomach: Nausea and vomiting with pains.

Stools: Jelly-like.

Extremities: Pains, contractions of hips and legs; sciatica.

Uses

1. Abdominal pain
2. Diarrhea
3. Indigestion
4. Nausea and Vomiting

XII. DULCAMARA
(Bitter Sweet)

Generalities

Often called the "wet remedy." Indicated for troubles which result from getting wet and chilled, or ailments made worse in damp, cold weather, especially at close of summer when days are warm and nights are cold; ill effects of sitting on cold, damp ground or getting chilled on a rainy day.

Modalities

Worse: Night; cold in general; damp, rainy weather.

Better: Moving around; external warmth.

Clinical Picture

Nose: Stuffy in cold dampness; alternating blocked and profuse discharge.

Throat: Thirst.

Abdomen: Pain around navel.

Stools: Green, watery.

Respiratory: Loose cough.

Feet: Very cold.

Uses

1. Hayfever
2. Respiratory infection
   a. Coughs and colds

XIII. GELSEMIUM SEMPERVIRENS
(Gelsemium) (Yellow Jasmine)

Generalities

Adopted for typical "flu" symptoms with drowsiness, grogginess, trembling, listlessness, dullness, heaviness. Problems often brought on by grief or bad news. Muscular weakness. Patient has no appetite or thirst. Symptoms slow in onset preceded by weakness, langour and desire to lie down. Upon waking, there is trembling and sense of heaviness. Mental sluggishness, relaxed, torpid state; very sensitive to emotional shock.

Modalities

Worse: Damp weather; before storms; bad news; thinking about ailment; 10:00 a.m.

Better: Bending forward; urinating; perspiration; open air.

Clinical Picture

Head: Dull, heavy ache; muscle soreness in neck and shoulders.

Eyes: Eyelids heavy.

Nose: Sneezing, running; fullness and pain at root of nose.

Tongue: Thick, yellowish, trembling.

Throat: Difficulty swallowing; sore, rough, burning throat; pain in ears when

	swallowing.
Stomach:	Absence of hunger or thirst.
Stool:	Cream-colored or tea-green colored diarrhea.
Respiratory:	Dry, sore cough.
Back:	Aching.
Skin:	Measles—before rash, helps bring rash out.
Fever:	Shaking; long, exhausting sweats; chills without thirst.

XIV. HEPAR SULPHURIS CALCAREUM
(Hepar Sulph) (Sulphate of Lime and Hahnemann's Calcium Sulphide)

Generalities

Usually indicated for persons with light hair, soft muscles, who are oversensitive mentally and physically; usually peevish, angry at slightest provocation and hypochondriacal. Very sensitive to cold drafts. Unhealthy skin.

Modalities

Worse:　Dry, cold winds; draft; tough; lying on right side.

Better:　Damp weather; warmth; after eating.

Clinical Picture

Ears:　Throbbing, buzzing.

Nose:　Soreness of nostrils; sneezes in cold winds.

Face:　Yellowish complexion.

Throat:　Feels as though plug or splinter is lodged when swallowing. Pain from throat to ear when swallowing.

Abdomen:　Pain in upper right side under ribs; worse with cough, breathing.

Respiration:　Choking, croupy, strangulating cough. Worse being uncovered or eating cold food. Wheezing.

Skin:　Unhealthy skin that forms ulcer

from small scratches.

Uses
1. Abscesses
2. Croup
3. Ear problems

XV. HYPERICUM PERFOLIATUM
(Hypericum) (St. John's Wort)

Generalities

Indicated if pain of injury radiates from initial site toward center of body. Very useful to relieve pain; helps heal injuries to nerve-rich areas (toes, fingertips). *Hypericum* is the *Arnica* of the spinal column. Falls on, or blows to the spine, particularly the tailbone (coccyx) respond to *Hypericum*. *Hypericum* ointment or lotion may be used in some skin wounds, particularly those that appear infected and where pain is associated with the area of injury.

Uses
1. Eye disorders
2. Injuries
   a. Wounds
      i.   Incised wounds
      ii. Lacerated wounds
      iii. Scratches and abrasions
   b. Bites, stings and puncture wounds
   c. Bruises
   d. Burns

XVI. IGNATIA AMARA
(Ignatia) (St. Ignatius Bean)

Generalities
Emotional state is of utmost importance; alternating moods change quickly; extreme nervousness with trembling inside. Ill effects of grief and anger. Especially suited for nervous, sensitive, overconscientious, excited, dark-haired women with gentle dispositions. A remedy of erratic, contradictory, paradoxical symptoms.

Modalities
Worse: Morning; coffee; external warmth.
Better: Change of position; hard pressure.

Clinical Picture
Head: Congestion after anger or grief; worse from smelling tobacco. Pain is as if nail were driven through head.
Throat: Feeling as if lump were in throat; difficulty swallowing; "globus hystericus."
Stomach: Sinking feeling; worse with deep breath.
Stool: Diarrhea from fright.
Respiratory: Hollow, spasmodic cough; sighing.

Uses
1. Headache
2. Indigestion
3. Respiratory infection
   a. Sore throat
4. Travel sickness

XVII. IPECACUANHA
(Ipecac) (Ipecac Root)

Generalities
Most indicated for complaints of persistent nausea not relieved by vomiting; ailments caused by eating rich or indigestible food such as ice-cream, sweets (compare with *Nux Vomica, Pulsatilla*).   Stout, fat people who catch cold easily; history of easy hemorrhaging.

Modalities
Worse: Warm, moist weather; lying down.

Clinical Picture
Eyes: Rings of blueness.
Tongue: Clean.
Stomach: Constant nausea and vomiting.
Abdomen: Flatulent; clutching pain around navel.
Throat: Thirstless.
Menses: Bright red blood, too long.
Respiratory: Asthma returning periodically; cough incessant with each breath; feels full of mucus but nothing comes up.
Stool: Greenish diarrhea, like frothy molasses.

Uses
1. Abdominal pain
2. Asthma
3. Bleeding
4. Diarrhea
5. Hoarseness
6. Indigestion
7. Nausea and vomiting

XVIII. LEDUM PALUSTRE
(Ledum) (Marsh Tea)

Generalities
Although it has other uses, *Ledum* for the Home Prescriber is used for stabs and puncture wounds from sharp, pointed instruments, from animal bites and from certain insect bites. It is for the particular pain associated with such wounds, particularly if wounded parts are cold yet pain is relieved by cold application. It follows *Arnica* well for cases of severe local bruising and black eyes which do not respond fully to *Arnica* (compare with *Hypericum*).

Uses
1. Eye disorder
2. Injuries
   a. Bites, stings, puncture wounds
   b. Bruises

XIX. MERCURIUS SOL
(Quicksilver)

Generalities
Indicated when trouble has already developed. Adapted for people who are very sensitive to heat or cold weather changes. Swollen glands; profuse sweat; bodily secretions often foul, including pus, sweat, breath; stools often loose. Thin, green-yellow discharges, often profuse and excoriating.

Modalities
Worse: Night; perspiration; wet, damp weather; lying on right side; warm bed.

Better: Bed rest.

Clinical Picture
Nose: Sneezing; nostrils raw, reddened by nasal discharge.

Mouth: Metallic taste; increased saliva; bad teeth; sharp, pulsating toothache, radiating to ears.

Throat: Sore; worse on right side.

Stomach: Intense thirst for cold drinks.

Stool: Green, bloody, slimy; painful; worse at night.

Respiratory: Cough with yellow-green sputum.

Skin: Constantly moist; glands swollen.

Uses
1. Diarrhea
2. Ear problems
3. Respiratory infection
   a. Coughs and colds
   b. Sore throat
4. Toothache

XX. NUX VOMICA
(Poison Nut)

Generalities
Remedy for overindulgence. Adapted especially to thin, irritable, zealous persons with dark hair—most often men; quarrelsome, nervous, intelligent, hypochondriacal; oversensitive to noise, music, light; craves stimulants.

Modalities
Worse:	Overeating; coffee; tobacco; mental overexertion.
Better:	Wet weather; lying down.

Clinical Picture
Head:	Aching, worse in sunshine; accompanied by irritable feeling.
Nose:	Dry, stuffy.
Tongue:	First half clean; posterior fur; white edges.
Throat:	Dry, scraped; worse in morning and in late evening, after overeating.
Stomach:	Nausea, worse in morning, after eating; sensitive to pressure.
Stool:	Constipation; ineffectual urge to pass stool.
Respiratory:	Asthma, worse with full stomach, overeating.

Dosage
Best given at night.

Uses
1. Abdominal pain
2. Asthma
3. Diarrhea
4. Hayfever
5. Headache
6. Hemorrhoids
7. Indigestion
8. Nausea and vomiting
9. Respiratory infection
   a. Coughs and colds
   b. Sore throat
10. Travel sickness

XXI. PULSATILLA NIGRICANS
(Pulsatilla) (Wood Flower)

Generalities

Remedy often best suited to women and children with blond or sandy hair and blue eyes; mild, gentle, timid, yielding and easily moved to laughter and tears, or men with similar characteristics. The *Pulsatilla* person craves sympathy and the company of others; moods changeable and fickle. (Mentally and physically, the direct opposite of *Nux Vomica* and *Chamomilla*). Patient is chilly, but averse to heat; responses are not sharp or intense, but suppressed, gradual, sluggish. Symptoms are erratic, change frequently. Most distinctive pains of *Pulsatilla* patient are wandering pains and pains that grow gradually in intensity. Fever without thirst despite dry mouth.

Modalities

Worse: Evening before midnight; warmth (room, applications or coverings); after eating fat, rich food.

Better: Open air; cold applications; consolation.

Clinical Picture

Ears: Sensation as if something were being forced outward; difficulty hearing, as if ears were stuffed.

Nose:	Yellow mucus abundant in morning; stoppage in evening.
Mouth:	Dry mouth without thirst.
Tongue:	Yellow or white, covered with tenacious mucus.
Stomach:	Averse to fat, warm food and drink. Vomits clear yellow liquid in morning, especially with morning sickness of pregnancy.
Respiratory:	Dry cough evening and night.

Uses
1. Chicken Pox
2. Ear problems
3. Fever
4. Headache
5. Indigestion
6. Measles
7. Mumps
8. Nausea and vomiting
9. Respiratory infection
   a. Coughs and colds
10. Styes
11. Toothache

XXII. RHUS TOXICODENDRON
(Rhus Tox) (Poison Oak)

Generalities

Patient is extremely restless; frequent change of position which temporarily improves pains and anxiety; characterized by sadness; mainly affects joints and their attachments (tendons and ligaments) causing tearing pains.

Modalities

Worse: Sleep; cold, wet weather; night; at rest.

Better: Change of position; warm, dry weather; warm applications; continued movement.

Clinical Picture

Face: Jaws crack; glands swollen and painful; mumps with restlessness.

Stomach: Nausea with dizziness from traveling.

Stool: Bloody, mucousy diarrhea.

Respiratory: Hoarseness from overusing voice; dry, teasing cough—more after midnight.

Extremities: Tearing pains in ligaments, tendons and muscles; swelling in joints; arthritic pains relieved by gentle motion; better with warm applications.

Skin: Itching with blisters; red; swollen
                 like Chicken Pox or Poison Ivy.

Uses
   1. Chicken Pox
   2. Diarrhea
   3. Hoarseness
   4. Injuries
      a. Sprains and strains
   5. Mumps
   6. Poison Ivy or Oak
   7. Respiratory infection
      a. Coughs and colds
   8. Travel sickness

XXIII. RUTA GRAVEOLENS
(Ruta) (Rue-Bitterwort)

Generalities
Used in sprains, after *Arnica*, when site of injury seems to be where tendons join the bone. Hard deposits may be formed at site of injury near bone.

Modalities
Worse: Cold, wet weather; lying; every motion of affected part (compare with *Rhus Tox*).

Clinical Picture
Eyes: Red; hot; painful after close work such as sewing; headache after eye strain.

Back and Extremities: Pain; bruised feeling in small of back and loins, hamstrings and Achilles tendon; lumbago; worse before rising.

Uses
1. Headache
2. Injuries
   a. Bruises
   b. Sprains and strains

XXIV. SPONGIA TOSTA
(Spongia) (Roasted Sponge)

Generalities
Used in symptoms of respiratory organs; cough, croup; anxiety and difficulty breathing. Exhaustion of body after slight exertion.

Modalities
Worse: Ascending; wind; cold; before midnight.
Better: Descending; head low.

Clinical Picture
Respiratory: Dryness of air passages; burning of larynx (voice box), which is sensitive to touch; feels as if plug is stuck there. Croup worse during inspiration and before midnight. Cough better after eating or drinking, especially warm drinks. Wheezing, worse in cold air with increased phlegm.

Uses
1. Croup
2. Respiratory infection
   a. Coughs and colds

XXV. STICTA PULMONARIA
(Sticta) (Lungwort)

Generalities
Used for respiratory symptoms: cough with head cold, runny nose; sneezing; joint pains often present.

Modalities
Worse: Sudden change of temperature; evening; inspiration.

Clinical Picture
Respiratory: Throat raw; post-nasal drip; cough dry, hacking during night.

Uses
1. Headache
2. Respiratory infection
   a. Coughs and colds

BIBLIOGRAPHY

Allen, H.C., M.D. *Keynotes and Characteristics of the Materia Medica with Nosodes.* Jain Publishing Co., New Delhi, India.

Baker, W. P., M.D., Neiswander, A.C., M.D., and Young, W.W., M.D. *Introduction to Homeotherapeutics.* American Institute of Homeopathy, Washington, D.C.; 1974.

Boericke, William, M.D. *Pocket Manual of Homeopathic Materia Medica with Repertory*, 9th Ed. Boericke & Runyon, Philadelphia, PA; 1927.

Cox, D. and Hyne-Jones, T.W. *Before the Doctor Comes.* Health Science Press. Rustington, Sussex, England; 1974.

Dewey, W.A., M.D. *Practical Homeopathic Therapeutics*, 3rd Ed., Jain Publishing Company, New Delhi, India.

Gibson, D.M., M.D. *First Aid Homeopathy in Accidents and Ailments*, 4th Ed. The British Homeopathic Association, London; 1975.

Kent, James Tyler, M.D. *Lectures on Homeopathic Materia Medica with New Remedies.* Jain Publishing Co., New Delhi, India.

Nash, E.B., M.D. *Leaders in Homeopathic Therapeutics*, 6th Ed. Boericke and Tafel, Philadelphia; 1926.

Shepherd, Dorothy, M.D. *Homeopathy for the First Aider*, 2nd Ed. Health Science Press. Rustington, Sussex, England; 1953.

BOOKS PUBLISHED BY THE HIMALAYAN INSTITUTE

Living with the Himalayan Masters	Swami Rama
Yoga and Psychotherapy	Swami Rama, R. Ballentine, M.D. Swami Ajaya
Emotion to Enlightenment	Swami Rama, Swami Ajaya
A Practical Guide to Holistic Health	Swami Rama
Freedom from the Bondage of Karma	Swami Rama
Book of Wisdom	Swami Rama
Lectures on Yoga	Swami Rama
Life Here and Hereafter	Swami Rama
Marriage, Parenthood and Enlightenment	Swami Rama
Meditation in Christianity	Swami Rama et al.
Superconscious Meditation	Pandit Usharbudh Arya, Ph.D.
Philosophy of Hatha Yoga	Pandit Usharbudh Arya, Ph.D.
Yoga Psychology	Swami Ajaya
Foundations of Eastern and Western Psychology	Swami Ajaya (ed)
Psychology East and West	Swami Ajaya (ed)
Meditational Therapy	Swami Ajaya (ed)
Diet and Nutrition	Rudolph Ballentine, M.D.
Theory and Practice of Meditation	Rudolph Ballentine, M.D. (ed)
Science of Breath	Rudolph Ballentine, M.D. (ed)
Joints and Glands Exercises	Rudolph Ballentine, M.D. (ed)
Yoga and Christianity	Justin O'Brien, Ph.D.
Inner Paths	Justin O'Brien, Ph.D. (ed)
Faces of Meditation	S. N. Agnihotri, Justin O'Brien (ed)
Sanskrit Without Tears	S. N. Agnihotri, Ph.D.
Art and Science of Meditation	L. K. Misra, Ph.D. (ed)
Swami Rama of the Himalayas	L. K. Misra, Ph.D. (ed)
Science Studies Yoga	James Funderburk, Ph.D.
Homeopathic Remedies	D. Anderson, M.D., D. Buegel, M.D., D. Chernin, M.D.
Hatha Yoga Manual I	Samskrti and Veda
Hatha Yoga Manual II	Samskrti and Judith Franks
Practical Vedanta	Brandt Dayton
The Swami and Sam	Brandt Dayton
Chants from Eternity	Institute Staff
Thought for the Day	Institute Staff
Spiritual Diary	Institute Staff
Himalayan Mountain Cookery	Martha Ballentine
The Yoga Way Cookbook	Institute Staff